STOP YOUR TINNITUS:

CAUSES, PREVENTATIVES, AND TREATMENTS

by Phyllis Avery

HYGEIA PUBLISHING COMPANY
1358 FERN PLACE
VISTA, CALIFORNIA 92083

This book is a reference work based on a literature search by the author. The suggestions are not intended to take the place of government-authorized medical care or as medical advice.

Published in the United States of America

Library of Congress Cataloging in Publishing 91-76653

Avery, Phyllis

Stop Your Tinnitus, Causes, Preventatives, and Treatments

ISBN 1-880598-22-1

Other books by Phyllis Avery:

The Garden of Eden Raw Fruit & Vegetable Recipes
The 10-Minute Vegetarian Cookbook
Stop Your Indigestion: Causes, Remedies, and Recipes

Address inquiries with a stamped, self-addressed envelope to:

Phyllis Avery
1358 Fern Place
Vista, CA 92083

Cover designed by Phyllis Avery

TABLE OF CONTENTS

INTRODUCTION

I am a 57-year-old woman who had tinnitus for five years and now seems free of it thanks to my determination to find and eliminate its root causes.

While doing the library research for this book, I came to understand for the first time the correlation between my tinnitus and the penicillin shot I was given for pneumonia at the age of three months. Babies under the age of one year have not developed an immune system to prevent bodily invasions by toxic substances. Unless the toxins acquired over time are eliminated by eating natural foods and by exercising to excrete them through the skin, they remain in the body.

Both of my parents smoked. We lived in New Jersey, so during the long winter months in a closed environment I was breathing cigarette smoke continuously. Scientists now recognize that side-stream smoke is as harmful as direct smoke. As a result of the polluted air of our home, I grew up as a sickly child, suffering from colds that kept me in bed several days every year. The doctors gave me antibiotics, which are known to destroy valuable white blood cells. In my late teens I developed allergies.

As a young woman I worked in the garment industry as a dress designer. The dress goods are coated with formaldehyde for the purpose of "sizing" the fabric—to keep it firm during production. The odor was so powerful that my eyes would fill with tears. I never considered that the formaldehyde was accumulating in my tissues and causing untold damage.

Twelve years after working in the garment industry, my husband and I bought a new townhouse. Formaldehyde was seeping out of the cabinets. Vapors from the new synthetic wall-to-wall carpeting were gassing out. The unit had a gas kitchen stove and its own gas furnace. The garage below housed my husband's diesel car. After six months of almost continuous health problems, I had a physical breakdown. A contributing factor surely was the stress from a lifetime of family problems.

My whole body went haywire. I was unable to eat some of the simplest of foods; most foods I couldn't digest or assimilate. I couldn't sleep. Everything made me nervous. I became a universal reactor—allergic to food, chemicals, and airborne particles. Tinnitus began intermittently, and later hounded me continuously.

As with many tinnitus sufferers, I have spent thousands of dollars and many hours in search of relief by visiting a variety of doctors and therapists. Since I was not benefiting from any of their treatments, I started a tinnitus self-help group in my area to compare notes with other sufferers and for emotional support. There are members in the group who have traveled as far as India and China because they had read about a recent breakthrough or a remedy unavailable in the United States. This book shares with you the experiences and newfound knowledge of the entire group.

Perhaps this book should be subtitled "Obsessed with Tinnitus." Because of my low tolerance for pain and discomfort, I was trying to rid myself of it by researching books and journals at medical libraries, talking to anyone who might know something about it, writing to people who reported experiences in health magazines, contacting doctors whose reports I read of in medical journals, going to a range of practitioners from acupuncturists to psychiatrists, experimenting with herbs, vitamins, devices, and various body positions, and trying all the therapies that seemed to be selectively benefiting others in the tinnitus group.

I've made the attempt here to share all the tinnitus-related information gathered by the group from medical journals, medical consultations, books, health newsletters, seminars, health magazines, science papers, and medical dictionaries. The more one knows about a particular malady, the better one can make intelligent decisions in attempting self-treatment and avoiding measures that could permanently damage the ear. And without an understanding of the causes of tinnitus, the sufferer will not be alerted to avoid the many everyday factors that exacerbate the problem and perpetuate the noise.

Although this book relates more to sufferers whose tinnitus is the result of temporary damage from environmental factors than to those whose hearing apparatus has been permanently damaged by percussive noises or head injuries, it has much to offer regardless of the cause of the problem.

Identifiable sources of information are referenced. As editor, I take full responsibility for the book's contents. It presents information presented by all group members. Even though I disagree with some of what is included, it is all retained so the reader can reach his/her own conclusions.

Tinnitus can be one of the most frustrating and irritating problems to live and deal with. Since there are over a hundred causes for the problem, a technique that corrects the condition for one person may do absolutely nothing for someone else. Correction is difficult in part due to the remarkable sensitivity of the ear.

I can tell you at the outset that ridding yourself of tinnitus caused by toxins, drugs, and chemicals is not going to be easy. You will not succeed without unwavering determination.

I would like to thank T.C. Fry of Health Excellence Systems for allowing me to use his organization's literature as long as proper credit is given.

I am also grateful to Lowel Ponte, a science journalist, who assisted me in editing this book.

HOW WE HEAR

Sound waves consisting of waves of pressure, are transmitted through the air, collecting in the outer ear, which helps direct sound waves into the ear canal. When they reach the ear drum, they cause it to vibrate. This vibration is passed on to the three bones of the middle ear, the malleus, incus and stapes, which are arranged in a chain and which transmit this vibration to the inner ear.

Sound vibrations are then transmitted through the inner ear which is filled with fluid. This transmits sound waves to the cochlea, which is shaped like a snail. Cells bristling with specialized hairs, which are sensitive to movement, are distributed along the length of the cochlea. As the waves pass, they are "sensed" as pressure, and transmitted along the cochlea nerve to the auditory area of the brain where they are interpreted. High frequency tones are sensed only by the specialized cells in the first part of the cochlea, whereas medium and low tones are sensed further along.

The way in which waves are turned into electrical energy and interpreted by the brain is not understood. The current theory is that the cells of the cochlea measure pressure waves in the endolymph and turn them into electrical impulses. See Figure 1.

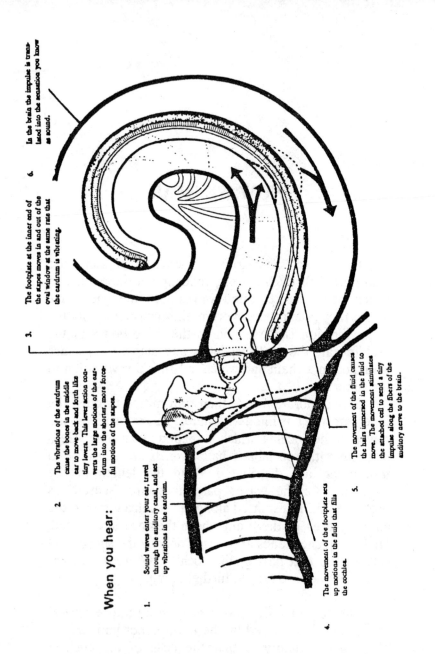

When you hear:

1. Sound waves enter your ear, travel through the auditory canal, and set up vibrations in the eardrum.

2. The vibrations of the eardrum cause the bones in the middle ear to move back and forth like tiny levers. This lever action converts the large motions of the eardrum into the shorter, more forceful motions of the stapes.

3. The footplate at the inner end of the stapes moves in and out of the oval window at the same rate that the eardrum is vibrating.

4. The movement of the footplate sets up motions in the fluid that fills the cochlea.

5. The movement of the fluid causes the hairs immersed in the fluid to move. The movement stimulates the attached cell to send a tiny impulse along the fibers of the auditory nerve to the brain.

6. In the brain the impulse is translated into the sensation you know as sound.

Figure 1. A SCHEMATIC DIAGRAM OF HOW THE HUMAN EAR FUNCTIONS.
Source: Quieting: A practical Guide to Noise Control.[10]

6

The fragile eardrum is protected by a muscle called the *tensor tympani,* which dampens dangerously loud noises, and by the *eustachian tube,* an opening that connects the middle-ear chamber with the open throat and allows equalization of the air pressure on either side of the eardrum. The semicircular canals in the area of the inner ear are non-auditory organs that control balance.[1]

Figure 2 is a general reference applicable to the entire text.

THE AUDITORY SYSTEM

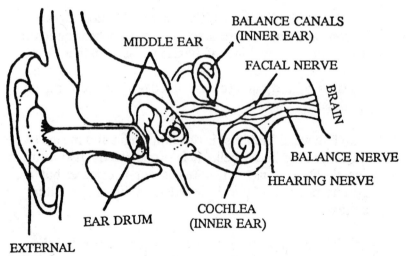

Figure 2. Source: American Tinnitus Association. Portland, Oregon.

WHAT IS TINNITUS?

Tinnitus is the term applied generally to noises that arise spontaneously in one or both ears. In different people—and in the same person at different times—it can range from barely audible to quite loud. Tinnitus is a symptom, often accompanied by other symptoms, experienced by those with hearing disorders. Most people with tinnitus report a high-pitched ringing; others a buzzing, hissing, roaring, whistling, chirping, crickets, or other sound, when in fact no such external physical sounds are present at the ear.

In the early stage of the malady, attacks of these extraneous sounds come and go—days, weeks, or months apart. In advanced stages the sound becomes constant—all day, all night.[2]

Lawrence E. Lamb, MD, writes that almost all cases of constant tinnitus are associated with a hearing loss. This can be any kind of hearing loss, whether from otosclerosis or other middle-ear problems. Many diseases of the ear are associated with some form of tinnitus.[3]

The word "tinnitus" is of Latin origin and means to tinkle or ring like a bell. It is pronounced TIN-nit-tus (or tin-NIGHT-us). Tinnitus is not a disease, but a symptom of a physical disorder within the auditory system.

Tinnitus may be classified as objective or subjective. Arthur S. Freese, in You and Your Hearing, explains as follows: In the former, the person hears an actual sound that is being generated within the body from somewhere outside the auditory system. When the sound is a

8

blowing kind and coincides with the sufferer's respiration, it indicates an abnormally open eustachian tube. When it is pulsating in rhythm with the heartbeat, it indicates an aneurysm (a weak spot in a blood-vessel wall). When it's a series of sharp regular clicks heard for a few seconds or minutes at a time, it's due to contractions of the muscles at the roof of the mouth.[4]

The Textbook of Medicine adds to the definition: objective tinnitus is usually caused by noises such as those from temporomandibular (jaw) joints, opening of eustachian tubes, or repetitive contraction of the stapedius muscle. When it's very quiet, a person may actually hear the pulsating flow of blood in his carotid arteries.[5]

Freese continues: Subjective tinnitus is heard by the sufferer only and is more frequently suffered due to damage of the hair cells, Ménière's Disease, ototoxic drugs, etc. Oddly enough, even when the acoustic nerve is cut (which has been done for Ménière's disease or in removing an acoustic neuroma) tinnitus often remains. This may indicate that the source of the sound lies in some malfunction of the acoustic nerve deep within the skull in the neural pathways that go from the acoustic nerve up to the auditory cortex.

Although tinnitus is a symptom of an inner-ear problem, and not of a serious disease, it should be checked by competent experts or it can lead to a total loss of hearing or "at least" to years of unnecessary misery.[4]

Subjective tinnitus can originate from anywhere in the auditory system, as explained in The Textbook of Medicine. The sounds most often complained of are buzzing, blowing, roaring, clanging, or popping.[5]

Deafness and tinnitus can result from exposure to certain chemicals connected with one's occupation, according to J. I. Rodale. These can be aniline, arsenic, benzene, mercury, lead, carbon monoxide, illuminating gas, phosphorus, and sulphur.

Rodale disagrees with Freese regarding the seriousness of tinnitus when he states that tinnitus and deafness often act as a clue to other serious systemic defects. Diabetes, inflammation of the kidneys, a faulty fat metabolism are three such conditions, and one should have one's blood examined for sugar, urea, and cholesterol levels if tinnitus occurs. Virus infections are also likely to result in this type of ear trouble.[6]

In 1986 the American Tinnitus Association, in Portland, Oregon, gleaned from nearly 5000 letters over the previous six years, information about what people felt had started their tinnitus. This compilation is not claimed to be all-inclusive or statistically accurate, but it does demonstrate the broad variety of factors that can cause tinnitus.

CAUSES ASCRIBED	NUMBER OF PEOPLE REPORTING
Hearing Loss	1253
Military Service	982
Noise	659
Accidents	418
Ménière's syndrome	362
Influenza	305
Ear Infection	202
Flying	176

Instant Hearing Loss	137
Dental Work	107
Heredity	97
Head Cold	86
Kidney Infection	62
Sinus Infection	43
Childbirth	36
Mumps	32
Swimming	28
Rheumatic Fever	18
Measles	16
Scarlet Fever	12
Diphtheria	8
Neck Exercise	6
Sneeze	2
Hit by Lightning	2^7

This book discusses these and other tinnitus-inducing causes and disorders and ways to avoid them, then gives a rundown of the various therapies—physiological, psychological, and alimentary—through which sufferers have found relief. One of my purposes for writing is to make you aware of what measures are available to help you cope with this bothersome affliction. The decisions are yours.

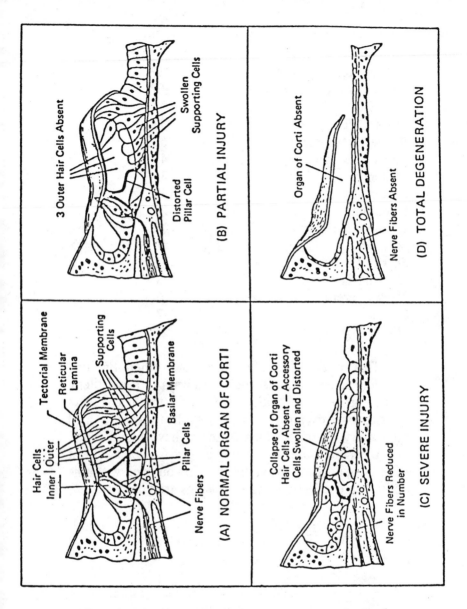

Figure 3. DRAWINGS OF THE HUMAN ORGAN OF CORTI
ARE SHOWN THAT ILLUSTRATE THE NORMAL STATE,
PANEL A, AND THE INCREASING DEGREES OF NOISE-
INDUCED PERMANENT INJURY, PANELS B, C, AND D.
Source: <u>Quieting: A Practical Guide to Noise Control</u>.[10]

12

EXTERNAL CAUSATIVE AGENTS

LOUD NOISES

Throughout history noise has exerted powerful influences on people, both good and bad. It has been used to frighten, to inspire, and to entertain. One belief held that the devil hated noise; hence church bells, bells on ships, the clinking together of glasses, and the general uproar associated with weddings were intended to drive away evil forces.

The industrial revolution brought advanced forms of mechanization, and noise became increasingly recognized as an occupational health hazard. Iron workers have repeatedly been cited as particularly vulnerable, and boiler making probably ranks as the supreme high risk skill among twentieth century observers dealing with occupational hearing loss.[8]

Sound is accompanied by vibrations. This is demonstrated by striking the prongs of a fork against a hard surface, and then touching the prongs to the ear. One can feel the vibrations of sound by pressing an ear against a radio speaker with the volume on high. The best way to demonstrate the vibration of sound is to press one's fingers against the front of the throat while speaking.

Sound can thus be defined as "a vibration that travels through suitable materials and to which human beings and animals may be sensitive."[9]

Loud noise is a health hazard. When you are in a sound field in which the level as read on a sound-level meter is 70 dB or more, even though you know consciously that you are in no danger, some part of your body tries to run away. The signs of this are the common symptoms of nervous stress: Your heart beats more quickly; breathing becomes shallower and faster; the pupils of your eyes dilate; the small blood-vessels in your skin contract; your blood pressure rises. These are actions of a body arousing itself to escape. During sleep the sound level need only exceed 55 dB to produce changes resembling the waking stress for 70 dB.[10]

You can become "accustomed" to the noises in your environment, but all that this means is that you can become accustomed to eliminating the noise from your conscious attention, just as the person who works all day around a bad odor soon ceases consciously to smell it. The physiological effects persist, however. If you are compelled to work in noisy surroundings, the only warnings of acoustically-induced stress may be signs of fatigue and nervous strain.

Noise damage to hearing is an insidious process. The immediate effects do not always indicate the ultimate results of exposure. Exposure to a mildly excessive noise level results in a temporary desensitization of the ear, the so-called "temporary threshold shift," a temporary loss of the ability to detect faint sounds. Noises likely to cause a temporary threshold shift are encountered during subway rides and airplane trips. Some degree of temporary threshold shift may be detectable even on the day following exposure, but ultimate recovery can be complete.

However, this pattern of threshold rise and recovery sometimes goes on through a number of cycles without any further evidence of damage, and then there may be a sudden failure to make complete recovery. This permanent effect is a sensorineural hearing loss.

One possible after-effect of exposure to an excessively intense noise is tinnitus, which seems to represent a spontaneous firing of signal impulses by the hair cells.[10]

Gunfire or an explosion causes irritation of the nerve endings of the inner ear. Sometimes the ringing from such acoustic trauma will be temporary, but it can last permanently, as it does with former President Ronald Reagan. He suffers to this day with concussion of a .38-caliber blank cartridge fired from a pistol held less than 6 inches from his ear more than 50 years ago on a movie set where he was acting.

From that moment in the 1930's, there has been a constant, unremitting ringing, like a telephone forever unanswered, sounding in the right ear of Ronald Reagan.[7a]

Sport hunters also suffer from acoustic trauma. The peak sound level from a 12-gauge shotgun has been measured between 140 dB to 165 dB. These intensity levels are damaging to the human cochlea. Acoustic trauma may be displayed by tinnitus, hearing loss, a full feeling in the ear, or pain. Recovery time varies from a few hours to several days depending upon the degree of trauma. Lack of recovery from severe damage is referred to as "noise-induced permanent threshold shift."[11]

Richard Carmen, tells us in his book <u>Our Endangered Hearing</u>, noise is defined as a "potentially damaging unwanted sound." The United States Public Health Service stated in early 1960, that hearing problems were the nation's most chronic handicapping disability. More people in the United States are afflicted with permanent hearing problems than are afflicted with blindness, multiple sclerosis, tuberculosis, kidney disease, liver disease, venereal disease and cancer <u>combined</u>.[12]

Freese adds that noise contributes to social violence, psychoses, neuroses, birth defects, and stress. Stress in turn leads to stress-related diseases including ulcerative colitis, rheumatoid arthritis, and high blood pressure, hypertension, diabetes, and peptic ulcer, cardiovascular injury, and stroke.[4, pp78-79]

Additional symptoms according to an assortment of newspaper articles, magazine columns, and news stories, include headaches, digestive problems, learning difficulties, irritability, insomnia, fatigue, reduced work efficiency, increased accidents and errors, suicide, and socially undesirable behavior. In men, research indicates that sound can increase sexual drive while diminishing sexual potency. In pregnant women, sound can alter the rate and form of fetal development.[editor]

Sound is measured in decibels, (dB) on a scale that increases logarithmically. Zero decibels (also known as the threshold level) is the lowest level of sound that a young human ear can detect. Compared with a 10-dB sound, a 20-dB sound wave has 10 times as much energy (and sounds about twice as loud); 30 dB has 100 times as much energy (and sounds about three times as loud), etc.[13]

The following table lists the approximate sound levels generated by some common sources, relative to threshold:

SOURCE	SOUND LEVEL, IN dB ABOVE THRESHOLD
Light Whisper	10
Quiet Conversation	20
Normal Conversation	30
Light Traffic	40
Typewriter, Loud Voices	50
Normal Traffic, Quiet Train	70
Vacuum Cleaner, Screaming Child	75
Dishwasher	75
Alarm-Clock Bell	80
Diesel Truck	80
Electric Shaver	85
Crowded School Bus	85
School Recesses/Assemblies	85
Pneumatic Drill (From 50 Feet)	90
Heavy Traffic, Thunder, Food Blender	90
High Speed Riding on Freeway in a Convertible	95
Newspaper Press	97
Farm Tractor	98
Garbage Truck	100
Lawn Mower, Chain Saw, Jackhammer, Subway	100
Unmuffled Motorcycle, Amplified Rock Music, Inboard Motorboat, Thunder, Sonic Boom, Riveting Machine	100
Threshold of Pain, Auto Horn	120
Air-Raid Siren	130
Snowmobile	135

Jet Airplane at Takeoff	140
Boom Unit in a Car	145
US Army Sergeant Rocket, Launched	
100 Feet Away	145+
Carrier Jet Operation	150
Rifle Shot	160
Bazooka Fired 1 Foot From the Ear	163
Noise Level Causing Death in	
Experimental Animals	175
Howitzer, at Crew Position	190

An article written for AUDIO, by Leigh Silverman, titled, "Loud Music & Hearing Loss," reports that repeated exposure to noise levels of 85 dB for more than eight hours could cause permanent hearing loss and/or tinnitus because the hair cells that pick up sound-induced pressure waves for transmission through nerve cells to the brain are destroyed by high levels of sound. According to Dr. Alvin Katz, surgeon director at the Manhattan Eye, Ear, and Throat Hospital, "Someone exposing themselves to fewer than 10 rock concerts would probably develop hearing loss." Dr. George Haspiel of St. Luke's Hospital in San Francisco agrees: "Kids exposed to rock music—their ears look very much like those of war veterans who have been exposed to artillery."

Two former rock musicians who can no longer perform due to tinnitus are Commander Cody and Chuck Stevens. Stevens has a physical intolerance to loud music. "Whenever I played," recalls Stevens, "pains would travel up my arms, into my neck, and into my ears." Bassist Jay Morse gave up playing when he began noticing aural discomfort during rehearsals. (His band rehearsed at levels up to 134 dB.) Now Morse's ears are so sensitive that he has to wear ear plugs when he walks down the street.[14]

Figure 1 also shows the process of how sounds arrive at your ear through the air reach the auditory nerve at the entrance to your brain. Like any well-engineered system, your ear has a few external protective devices. If you are exposed to an excessively loud noise, the muscle tensing your eardrum pulls taut, desensitizing it. This "stapedius reflex" takes place at sound levels between 80 and 95 dB. The point of onset of the reflect varies with individual sensitivity. Some persons can operate the stapedius reflex at will; from their experience it is evident that the desensitization is of the order of 20 dB. Thus the protection afforded by the stapedius reflex is important.[10, p9]

However, a burst of intense sound pressure too abrupt to give the stapedius reflex time to act can occur. In that event, the drum membrane is likely to rupture, causing a temporary loss of hearing and a hazard of middle ear infection. Since it is sometimes necessary to lance the drum membrane, subsequently forming scar tissue, any ear infections must be attended to at once to avoid a residue of permanent loss.

"Loud noise wears down the delicate hair cells in the inner ear, which translate sound into nerve impulses. If the noise is really high, as in an explosion, it can destroy the hair cells outright. At slightly lower levels -- a rock concert, for instance, or a noisy industrial job -- the damage is slow but steady." See Figure 3. Exposure to excessively intense noise is likely to cause tinnitus which represents a spontaneous firing of signal impulses by the hair cells.[10, p10]

Carmen notes that headphones/earphones shaped to fit one or both ears are widely used by telephone operators, radio and television engineers, musicians in

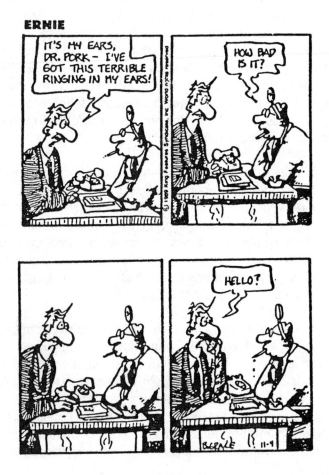

Reprinted with special permission of
King Features Syndicate, Inc.

recording studios, airplane pilots, etc. Listening to any stimulus through a headphone reduces the source distance to less than two inches. Sound from a loudspeaker is reflected or absorbed by everything in its path, such as draperies, carpeting, furniture, and even people; but transmitted from an earphone, it impinges only upon the ear parts, with nothing else to absorb it. Therefore, a sound level of 85 dB at an earpiece is far more hazardous than the same level at a loudspeaker in a well-furnished room.[12]

Heavy ear protectors can give protection from loud noises. Used mostly in certain industrial environments, such headgear is not practical for widespread use to protect the ears from traffic noises, loud music, and vacuum cleaners. A product that is not too cumbersome to use, however, is Sleepwell Ear Stops.* They are made of cotton wool soaked in paraffin. You warm and thereby soften them up by rubbing them between your palms. They will then conform to the shape of your ear canal and reduce noise by 20 to 30 dB. This product is found in most drug stores or can be obtained from the supplier.[editor]

Sleep Shade Company*

*Each item so marked throughout this book is listed, along with the address or the name and address of the suppliers, under **RESOURCES.**

Simple insert-type ear protectors are usable where perhaps 10-20 dB of protection is sufficient to eliminate the chance of hearing loss. In general, these are more effective for high-frequency sounds such as whistles rather than for low-frequency sounds such as machinery noise or jet turbulence.[9, p12]

Really effective protection is offered by over-the-ear muffs, which look like a relatively large pair of headphones. For maximum protection, both muffs and inserts may be worn. Even the combination of muffs and ear protectors, however, can offer little more than 40 dB protection, for sound can enter the body by other paths, entering via the chest cavity, the throat, and the bones of the head.[9, p12]

Custom-made ear molds provide less attenuation (usually 15 dB), but they are designed specially for your ear and therefore can provide maximum comfort. While no plug can deter sound from entering your ear via skull bone or tissue, custom ear molds are designed so that the plug does not vibrate within the ear canal, thereby transmitting the vibrations to the cochlea.[14, p81]

If you are working in a noisy environment, wear protective devices. Look under Guns in the Yellow Pages. Earmuffs (ear defenders) must fit in order to shut out sounds and must be kept clean to prevent infection. Most types give about 40 to 50 dB of protection. Use both plugs and muffs when shooting firearms.[editor]

One available earplug is made of a soft, foam like material that can be rolled into a small cylinder and placed in the ear, where it then expands. It can reduce noise up to 50 dB at some frequencies. The product is named N.R.R. II, and is sold by Zee Medical, Inc.*

Evaluate your hobbies and lifestyle. Recreational vehicles, appliances, and even children's toys can sometimes be loud enough to damage hearing. Make your home a refuge for your ears. The hearing mechanism can tolerate noise much better if it gets a rest from continuous exposure. Install carpeting to absorb noise, place foam pads under blenders and mixers, and install vibration mounts under your dishwasher.

Note: Using the telephone during a thunderstorm could pose a hazard. Nearby lightening may induce high-level static in the telephone lines and produce a very loud pop in the earpiece.[15]

TOXINS AND DRUGS

This section may be the most important in the book. We are exposed to chemicals in our work places (copy machines, formaldehyde, ink), our food (preservatives, artificial colors and flavors, pesticides), our drinking water, our homes (cleaning agents, furniture polish, room deodorants, synthetic carpeting, vinyl floors and shades, perfumes). My doctor said of perfume, "If you won't drink it, don't breathe it." Cigarette smoking, alcoholic beverages, and the increased use of narcotics have brought on a plethora of physical and mental maladies.[16]

The combination of various medications within the body may act to produce hearing problems, but if taken independently may not be harmful. It has been generally agreed that the hair cells of the inner ear are the primary target of ototoxicity (hearing loss due to medication), while nerve degeneration is secondary.[12, p65]

There are a considerable number of ototoxic (ear-poisoning) drugs and chemicals that can produce hearing loss and tinnitus, either temporary or permanent. Since tinnitus is so often associated with hearing loss and usually precedes it, this symptom must be regarded with very marked concern should it appear. Toxins such as those in the rest of this section and under CHEMICALS, can cause sensorineural deafness.[12-p161, 4-p106, 16, 17]

ALCOHOL

Carmen states that alcohol is a known ototoxic drug. It is quite common to find hearing loss in heavy drinkers, in addition to complaints of tinnitus.[12, p65]

According to Earl Mindell's Vitamin Bible, alcohol is not a stimulant, but actually a sedative-depressant of the central nervous system. It is capable of rupturing veins. It destroys brain cells by causing the withdrawal of necessary water from them. Only four drinks a day are capable of causing organ damage.[18]

Paavo Airola, Ph.D., N.D., claims in his book How To Get Well; that alcoholics suffer from malnutrition and nutritional deficiencies due to over-processed and refined nutritionless foods. Nutritional deficiencies are the precursor of such alcoholism-predisposing conditions as hypoglycemia, adrenal insufficiency, chronic fatigue, craving for a "lift"—sweets, snacks, drinks, etc. Overindulgence creates a vicious cycle by further depleting the body of vitamins and leading to severe deficiencies in B-complex vitamins, zinc and magnesium. The body must be returned to optimum health to end the craving for alcohol.

When alcoholics are put on a 10—14 day cleansing juice fast with special supplements, cravings for alcohol are greatly reduced. This gives a good two-week start toward breaking the drinking habit. It is recommended that a substitute drink be taken such as a glass of fresh

24

fruit juice. When fresh fruit juice is unavailable, almonds, pumpkin and sunflower seeds, fresh fruit, etc. can provide a needed lift.[19]

Roger J. Williams, in Nutrition Against Disease explains that alcoholism might be caused by malnutrition of the brain cells. True alcoholism appears when malnutrition of the brain cells becomes severe. The steps to becoming an alcoholic are a gradual process.

Williams states, "I assert that no one who follows good nutritional practices will ever become an alcoholic."

Alcohol consumption, at high levels, undoubtedly acts in several ways to damage brain cells: stopping blood flow; direct or indirect poisoning of the brain cells; deprivation of the brain cells of minerals, amino acids, and vitamins by substituting naked calories for good food.

Williams makes dietary recommendations for the recovering alcoholic: whole grains, raw nuts and seeds, fresh fruits, and raw vegetables. For the all-important amino acids, eat high protein foods such as lean meats, fish, eggs, and cheeses. Recommended nutrients are glutamine, magnesium, and niacinamide. Foods to be omitted are all processed foods, white sugar, and white flour. Refined carbohydrate foods should largely be avoided.[20]

Examples of refined carbohydrates are breakfast cereals, white bread, instant potatoes, polished rice, white sugar, and pasta. Examples of complex carbohydrates are whole grains, corn, brown rice, squash, pumpkin, potato, pepper, carrots, and fruits.[editor]

An outstanding diet is Dr. Cooper's Fabulous Fructose Diet because it satisfies the sugar craving alcoholics have.[21]

Cooper offers two types of diets. One is a "Transition Diet," which uses fructose in artificial forms as found in special chewing gums, tablets, and syrups. The second is a "Permanent Diet" which relies on fresh fruits.

The tinnitus group has found that staying with natural foods is best.

Alcohol destroys digestive enzymes in the stomach and necessary natural flora in the intestinal tract.[22] Two former alcoholics in the group were instructed by their doctors, in order to restore the flora, to take Lactobacillus acidophilus. A product named Prima-Dophilus is enteric, meaning having a coating that allows it to pass unaffected through the harsh stomach acids that destroy acidophilus.

A highly recommended book for detoxing the body is, Detox.[23]

ANTIBIOTICS

Various antibiotics belonging to the family of aminoglyocides are considered ototoxic, meaning they can damage the structures and function of the ear. Neomycin, kanamycin, dihydrostreptomycin, and vancomycin primarily damage hearing, attacking the hair cells of the cochlea and causing a loss of ability to discriminate high tones. Once it occurs, the loss worsens with prolonged use of the drug and is irreversible.

Streptomycin and gentamycin cause destruction of the hair cells of the balancing organs.[24]

Mindell lists the possible side effects of taking antibiotics: nausea, diarrhea, vomiting, rectal or genital itching, vaginal discharge, stomach cramps, brown or black discoloration of tongue, sensitivity to sunlight, excessive thirst, increased urination, decreased urination, hives, and bruising of skin.[18, p61]

In another chapter about children's medicines, Mindell warns that antibiotics rob children of potassium.[18, p189]

Freese declares antibiotics such as streptomycin, kanamycin, gentamycin, and neomycin can cause permanent damage to the ear based on susceptibility to the drug. The damage may involve degeneration of the cochlear hair cells themselves.[4, p107]

T. C. Fry, a natural hygienist and director of Health Excellence Systems, related an interesting story about his refusal to be administered antibiotics. When you suffer a cut, burn or abrasion, a physician will routinely administer an antibiotic "to prevent infection" because without it the puffiness and pus that characterizes what is called infection will appear.

The medical rationale is that bacteria invade the site of the injury and cause the pus and swelling. Antibiotics supposedly destroy the bacteria.

Fry's knee was gashed about two inches after he ran and fell on a gravel road. The compound where he was staying had two MD's who insisted on administering antibiotics and closing the cut with stitches. He refused and asked only that the cut be cleaned with clean water and a bandage applied.

The bandage was changed daily with no sign of "infection" appearing. By the ninth day the scab came off, leaving a bright pink scar.

Fry explained to the physicians that he used to get "infections" like everyone else. But after detoxifying his body and keeping it pure by eating raw fruits and vegetables, exercising, getting adequate sleep and so on, there is no "morbid matter" in his body that needed to be eliminated in an extraordinary manner. If bacteria entered the body, they would be attacked by the defensive white blood cells.

The body uses injuries as outlets for its pent-up uneliminated wastes and morbid materials. The body transports the noxious substances to the wound site so that drainage can be more easily effected.

Fry pointed out that no "infection" occur when antibiotics are administered because the body is devitalized by them. Antibiotics are quite toxic and destroy billions of white blood cells which attempt to apprehend them for expulsion. Because of this new engaging and vitality-sapping body eliminative activity (that is, the getting rid of the antibiotics by the body's white blood cell complement), its energies are diverted from gathering and transporting uneliminated morbid materials for expulsion at the injury site as it usually does.[25]

ANTICANCER CHEMOTHERAPEUTIC AGENTS

A clinical report of ototoxicity associated with cisplatin therapy is in the journal, Cancer. The experiments were made on female cancer patients. Twenty-three of 31 patients developed hearing loss and 21 patients reported the onset of tinnitus.

Transient, high-pitched tinnitus was described by most patients. Some patients first noticed tinnitus after the first treatment, but others did not report it until after two or more treatments.

Sixteen of 21 patients who developed tinnitus also demonstrated hearing loss. Two patients who developed constant tinnitus demonstrated significant high-frequency hearing loss.[26]

In the book, The Conquest of Cancer, Dr. Virginia Livingston-Wheeler and Edmond G. Addeo, express their disdain for chemotherapy. Chemotherapy introduces certain highly toxic chemicals into the patient's system in the hope that they'll attack the tumor and kill it before it kills the patient... It is well known that the effect of certain chemotherapeutic drugs on the immune system is so severe that new areas of cancer may appear during or soon after the treatment designed to eradicate the old cancer. Finally, irradiation and chemotherapy patients often have their immune systems so destroyed that they contract infectious diseases, such as pneumonia, from which they die before the cancer has a chance to kill them... There is a great deal of important new work being done that can save millions of lives, and yet much of it is being politically suppressed.[27]

You may be wondering what the previous paragraphs

have to do with tinnitus. I want to emphasize the point that if the scientific community cannot find a "cure" for cancer, they are not likely to cure tinnitus. Some doctors are such strong believers in drugs, that they administer them without recognizing their harmful side effects. If you want to stop your tinnitus, you are going to have to research the topic and be able to discuss a variety of the modalities your doctor prescribes.

There are at least four clinics in Mexico that specialize in controlling and reversing some forms of cancer. Their residential treatment programs are comprehensive, combining attitudinal-motivational interventions with natural detoxification and rejuvenation therapies. Treatment programs are custom-tailored to each individual. Each client engages in an intensive detoxification program that includes supervised fasting, colonics, and sweat baths. As the toxins are released from the body, therapies to reverse cell degeneration and stimulate rejuvenation are implemented. These clinics are listed under "Resources."

Natural therapeutic techniques, depending on the client's condition, may include lymphatic massage, chelation, acupressure/acupuncture, ultrasound, hydrotherapy, live cell analysis, color and magnetic therapies, vitamins, herbs, bioelectrical medicine, homeopathic remedies, blood crystallization tests, iridology analysis, and a vegetarian nutrition program.

Clients stay at the clinic in semiprivate and private rooms for an average of two to four weeks. Treatment is continued at home for one year, with constant monitoring by the clinic.

Several people in our tinnitus group have been to the

American Metabolic Institute* in San Antonio, Mexico, for treatment of <u>Candida albicans</u> (a yeast infection). They saw cancer patients being carried in and watched them progress remarkably in a matter of days, seeing them walk out and go home in three to five weeks. This clinic has a US office through which it can be contacted.

I also recommend two books about cancer:

<u>Are You A Candidate for Cancer?</u>[25a]

<u>The Apocalyptics:</u>
<u>Cancer and the Big Lie.</u>[28]

CAFFEINE

Mindell states that caffeine is not only a powerful drug, but also excessive intake can cause benign breast disease and prostate problems, hypertensive heart disease, cancer of the bladder, heart attacks, appetite loss, weight loss, irritability, insomnia, feelings of flushing, chills, low fevers, birth defects, nervousness, and interference with DNA replication.[18, p210]

This stimulant is found in coffee, tea, cola drinks, chocolate, and over-the-counter drugs. Drip coffee contains 146 mg per cup. Coca-Cola contains 64 mg in a 12-ounce bottle. Excedrin contains 65 mg per pill. (Excedrin PM has no caffeine, but does have an antihistamine.)

To break the caffeine habit, taper off gradually. Start by mixing half-regular and half-decaffeinated coffee. Change your mug for a smaller cup. Sip the brew slowly or with a spoon. Dilute it with hot water or low-fat milk.

For a needed lift in the morning, there are several brands of herbal tea made for that purpose. Morning Upper is one, and Celestial Seasonings offers several varieties. Some people use cola drinks for a morning boost, but these drinks contain chemicals that may cause the tinnitus to flare up. In place of such worthless liquid, you might choose something of value like fresh fruit or vegetable juices. The fructose in two oranges first thing in the morning gives me a mental lift. The same reasoning holds true for chocolate: eat a piece of fruit instead of something that you can not be certain is caffeine-free.[editor]

If you taper off from coffee rather than stop cold turkey, you are unlikely to get severe withdrawal symptoms. Quitting should provide almost immediate relief from jangled nerves, but you may experience one or more of the following: headache, tremors, irritability, tiredness, lethargy, anxiety, depression. Any symptom can last from a day to two weeks. Avoid exercise and heavy work, which will aggravate a headache; sleep when you feel drowsy. If concentration is difficult, it may take several weeks to do detailed work.[23, p118]

Many of the recommendations under "Nicotine" are applicable to caffeine as well.

CLINICAL DRUGS

Clinically used substances such as Novocaine, Marcaine, chloroform, and iodine can be just as invasive as prescription drugs, and the comments above apply here as well.[editor]

A book that exposes the myths and fallacies about

32

drugs, and the comments above apply here as well.[editor]

A book that exposes the myths and fallacies about prescription drugs is Medical Drugs on Trial-Verdict Guilty, by Sidhwa. It is available from Health Excellence Systems.[25b]

Also, the book, Detox, is applicable to clinical drugs.[23]

Carmen states that certain drugs may be harmful to hearing. People who have a propensity for tinnitus should avoid them since loss of hearing is frequently the precursor of tinnitus.[12, p161]

The information of the products in which these drugs are found is from, A Consumer's Dictionary of Cosmetic Ingredients.[29]

Antipyrine. Used as an antiseptic in eye lotions, an antipyretic (anti-itch) component in skin preparations, and as an analgesic.[29, p33]

Camphor. Used in emollient creams, hair tonics, eye lotions, after-shave lotions, and skin lotions.[29, p52]

Chloroform. Used as a solvent for fats, oils, waxes, resins, and as a cleansing agent.[29, p61]

Iodine. Used as an antiseptic and germicide in cosmetics.[29, p126]

Neomycin. Used in underarm deodorants. Highly toxic to the eighth nerve, which involves hearing, and to the kidneys.[29, p151]

"DESIGNER DRUGS"

Michelle McCormick has explained what designer drugs are in her book, Designer-Drug Abuse. Originally, the phrase "designer drugs" referred to newly created drugs of abuse

33

drugs of abuse whose chemical structure had not been defined under the law. Because the law did not precisely describe these drugs, they were actually legal. They had been designed specifically for abuse, and for circumventing the law.

The law has been changed to close this loophole. These drugs fall into three categories: amphetamines, hallucinogens, and narcotics. Their street names include fentanyl, methamphetamine, ecstasy, LSD, and PCP.[30]

Designer drugs are renowned for their effects on consciousness and personality, and for the bizarre mental disturbances which they can induce. The way in which the drugs affect the brain's operation is simply not known, though it is clear that their chemical constituents disrupt cerebral microphysiology in some way.[31]

Withdrawal symptoms are torturous during the first 24 to 72 hours. The addict experiences a range of agonies including intestinal cramps, involuntary muscle spasms, vomiting, diarrhea, sweats, and depression.[30, pp34-35]

Follow the recommendations under "Nicotine" to detoxify these drugs from your system.

DIURETICS

An article in FDA CONSUMER, by Vern Modeland, states that the side effects of furosemide, a potent diuretic prescribed for people who have very severe kidney damage, has been found to cause tinnitus and transitory hearing impairment.[32]

M. S. Pathy has written a report titled, "The Use,

Action and Side Effects of Diuretics," in which he states that tinnitus and transient deafness has occurred with ethacrynic acid (a type of diuretic).

Pathy goes on to enumerate some of the side effects caused by several types of diuretics under certain conditions and dosage: nausea, vomiting, diarrhea, stomach inflammation, colitis, anorexia, elevated serum aric acid, acute attacks of gout, increased urinary calcium excretion, acute hemorrhaging of the pancreas, low sodium ions, incontinence of urine, abnormal increase in size of male breasts, rashes, potassium depletion, coma, and death.[33]

Paul Yanick, Jr., PhD, explains in an article titled, "Nutrition Can Help Your Hearing," that the sensory cell portion of the inner ear needs a combination of about 40 nutrients in the right proportions and working together to effectively deliver complete electrical information to the brain.

The chief elements found in this electrochemical environment are sodium and potassium, and they must be in specific ratios for optimal transmission. When there are nutrient deficiencies, insufficient blood flows via the small vessels feeding the cells of the inner ear.[34]

Cooper states that diuretics are drugs that cause a loss of body water and consequently a temporary loss of weight, but not a loss of body fat. Body fat is unaffected, but there is a loss of potassium, magnesium, and other substances needed by the body.[21, p167]

Nathan Pritikin goes on to say in The Pritikin Permanent Weight-Loss Manual that diuretics cause temporary weight loss only because they deplete the tissues of water—water needed for the normal functioning of all the cells of the body. When diuretics are discontinued, weight usually increases to more than what it was before taking the pills. This kind of drug is especially dangerous if combined with a high-protein diet that itself causes dehydration.[35]

Fry points out that diuretics work by stimulating the kidneys to draw water from the blood and excrete it in the urine. (Caffeine is a diuretic, which explains how coffee stimulates urination).

The most commonly used chemicals for diuresis are the thiazides, states Fry. The best known is Diuril. Other common thiazides are Hydro Diuril, Esidrix, Anhydron, Oretic and Enduron.

Thiazides can dehydrate you and cause nausea, weakness and drowsiness. They also rid the body of potassium, along with water, and can worsen diabetes.

Fry goes on to say that all diet drugs are unhealthfully dangerous, and should not be used on a sensible weight loss program. To attain ideal weight, raw, ripe fruits with some vegetables, nuts and seeds should be eaten.[25c]

HALLUCINOGENIC DRUGS

Marijuana, cocaine, morphine, and heroin typify these drugs.

Dennis McFadden wrote in his book, <u>Tinnitus, Facts, Theories, and Treatments</u>, that tinnitus is sometimes mentioned as a concomitant to cocaine use, and its vasoconstrictive actions make this claim believable. He also claims that marijuana can markedly increase a pre-existing tinnitus.[36]

Marijuana has some medical benefits in alleviating the nausea associated with cancer chemotherapy as well as in arresting the inner eye pressures of glaucoma, according to The Encyclopedia of Psychoactive Drugs: Marijuana. Unfortunately marijuana smoke has at least as many cancer-causing substances as tobacco smoke. Chronic users develop lung problems similar to those of cigarette smokers.

This reference points out that marijuana is psychologically addictive and may contain harmful molds, bacteria, and traces of paraquat, a herbicide that is lethal to humans if swallowed in doses as small as one-tenth ounce.

Not only does marijuana increase the amount of blood the heart has to pump, it also alters the body's immune system. This is the system which protects people against viruses, bacteria, and other infections, and plays a major role in preventing the growth and distribution of cancerous cells throughout the body.

Marijuana use can disturb a woman's menstrual cycle. Failure to ovulate normally results in unpredictable periods or infertility. Just as certain drugs cause mutations in the genetic material of the body, heavy marijuana use may cause increased chromosome breakage and damage.

Offspring of marijuana users may weigh less and be shorter than normal at birth. Marijuana is secreted in breast milk and may be toxic to the nursing infant.

When a heavy marijuana user quits smoking, he may suffer from one or more of the following: insomnia, loss of appetite, weakness, irritability, sweating, depression, anxiety, abdominal cramps, nausea, aching muscles, and slight tremors. These symptoms last for up to one week after the person stops smoking, and then decrease more slowly for up to one month or more.[22a, pp59-67]

In another book of the same series titled, Cocaine, the authors write that cocaine is used in local anesthetics since it is a vasoconstrictor (narrows or constricts blood vessels). Cocaine's prolonged anesthetic action allows long and otherwise painful surgery of the nose to be easily performed.

Cocaine abuse has many detrimental effects on the mind and body; it interferes with nerve transmission to the brain; reduces desire for food and water; increases respiration rate and body temperature; induces vomiting; causes tremors and convulsions at high doses; and can cause cardiac arrest, insomnia, paranoia, delusions of persecution, hallucinations, and cerebral hemorrhage.

Constant snorting damages the nasal membranes and causes nosebleeds and tender, irritated nostrils, along with anxiety, confusion, hostility, and cold sweats.[22b, pp32-37]

I am emphasizing the effects of using these drugs because even though by themselves they will cause tinnitus, the illnesses will lead to many medical drugs that will add to the toxic overload.

Most of the same comments can be said of morphine and heroin. Withdrawal symptoms are similar to marijuana.

38

Follow the recommendations under "Nicotine" to break free of these drugs.

NICOTINE

This main drug in cigarettes is a known vasoconstrictor. It inhibits the flow of blood throughout the body by narrowing the blood vessels, including those nourishing the ear. Ear surgery such as reconstruction of a new eardrum has statistically higher failure rates among people who smoke.[12, p65]

More than 90 percent of cigarette smoke is composed of lethal gases, mainly carbon monoxide, hydrogen cyanide, and nitrogen oxides. Furthermore, some 4600 other chemicals are found in the tar—the residue left in the filter and lungs after the smoke passes through.[23, p53]

Exposure to cigarette smoke in the household can cause chronic middle ear disease and related hearing problems in children, according to Michael J. Kraemer, MD, at Seattle Children's Orthopedic Hospital and Medical Center. They report that exposure to two or more household cigarette smokers increases the risk of persistent middle-ear fluid build-up by nearly three times.

Their study showed that smoke is most dangerous for children who have frequent nasal congestion or a tendency to certain allergies.

The report reveals that each year in the United States over one million operations are performed to insert tubes in children's ears to alleviate middle-ear infection. If left untreated, middle-ear problems can lead to hearing loss as well as difficulties with learning, speech, and behavior.[37]

John Waldrop and Janice McCall Failes report in Natural Health and Wellness Encyclopedia that women smokers have their menopause an average of two years earlier than non-smokers. The decreased estrogen leads to osteoporosis, increasing the risk of broken hips and collapsed vertebrae.[38]

S. S. Field wrote an article in READER'S DIGEST titled "Nicotine: Profile of Peril" reporting that among the potentially deadly emissions of cigarette tobacco are at least 7 known and a large number of suspected carcinogens. There are also 15 to 20 volatile substances which are either irritants or poisons.[39]

Nicotine is highly addictive. The craving is caused by the body's dependence on the substance, and the dependence increases with prolonged use. The body constantly eliminates toxins and poisons; so when the level of poison is reduced in a physiologically addicted person, the addict seeks another "fix" and the cycle continues.[31, 16:1668]

One way to stop this vicious cycle is to cleanse the body of the accumulated poisons. This can be done by a 10- to 14-day juice diet. During such a diet most toxins will be effectively excreted, most tissues cleansed and freed from the poison; the blood will be nearly purified, and most of the craving will disappear. After the juice diet, a 100 percent health-building diet of natural foods—unrefined, whole, and poison-free—must be maintained. Airola gives detailed juice diet instructions in his book, How To Get Well.[19, p153]

Mindell recommends vitamins A, C, and E, plus selenium to help overcome withdrawal symptoms from nicotine while trying to stop smoking.[40]

Withdrawal from nicotine can be eased by a prescription drug called Nicorette, which slowly releases a measured dose of nicotine into the body to reduce physical craving for tobacco products.

Another method is to take a half teaspoon of bicarbonate of soda in a glass of water two or three times daily. This sodium salt holds nicotine in the system and helps reduce withdrawal symptoms by giving the body more time to adapt to withdrawal. WARNING: This is unsafe for those on low sodium diets.

Association with non-smokers and regular aerobic exercise such as running, fast walking, tennis, swimming, bicycling, and hard physical labor help you give up smoking and resist the temptation to return to it.[editor]

The American Lung Association of San Diego and Imperial Counties in California, has produced an impressive 16-page tabloid titled, Freedom From Smoking. It is a step-by-step program designed to make quitting easier for the smoker. Apparently it was written by ex-smokers, because all of the physical and psychological roadblocks are examined and addressed. There are daily charts for you to follow, diet suggestions and ways to handle relapses.[41]

MUNICIPAL DRINKING WATER

Tap water can contain some or all of the following

substances: nitrates and nitrites, chlorides, fluorides, arsenic, barium, cadmium, chromium, lead, mercury, nickel, silver, copper, benzene, asbestos, carbon tetrachloride, chlorine, DDT, dioxin, toluene, vinyl chloride, and formaldehyde. All are poisonous to the body if present in excessive amounts. Excessive fluorides, for example, speed up the aging process, disarm the immune system, mottle the teeth, degenerate the bones, and cause cancer and genetic damage. It is one job of municipal water authorities to see that none of these elements occurs in excess.[42]

The majority of these chemicals are harmful to the ear.

Nevertheless, if you aren't satisfied with the potability of water in your area, you can buy bottled water or a filter system that purifies your drinking and cooking water. There are differences of opinion about which type of water to buy or which type of filtering system is best.[editor]

The New Natural Healing Encyclopedia has explained what the labels designate on bottled water. Don't look at the brand name, like "Spring Valley." Read the ingredients. The FDA regulates bottled water.

Spring Water: The FDA requires that it come from a deep underground source that flows naturally to the surface.

Natural Water: This can be ordinary tap water, city water that is filtered or treated some way before bottling. It probably has chlorine in it, and may have other minerals added or removed during the processing.

Club Soda: This is just tap water that has artificial carbonation added to it, as well as mineral salts for flavor. It probably has been filtered.

Seltzer: Same as club soda, except it has no mineral salts added. Usually it's also salt free.

Sparkling Water: May be either naturally or artificially carbonated.

Distilled or Demineralized Water: This is water that is processed by distillation or osmotic filtration to remove its mineral and dissolved material content.

Mineral Water: The FDA is unable to regulate this kind of bottled water because a national standard can not be made due to the variations of mineral content in local water.

Opponents of bottled spring water claim that it can contain a significant level of pollutants. They recommend using distilled water instead, and taking mineral supplements. Its proponents, on the other hand, claim that the minerals in the water are not only natural but also in the proper proportions.

One type of filter system uses a charcoal carbon filter and costs from $300 to $600. After reading the literature on the many filter systems and comparing the facts, I recommend the reverse osmosis type.

Three national companies that offer reverse osmosis water systems are Amway, Shaklee, and Culligan. Two other companies offer excellent systems:

Nigra Enterprises and
Nature's Sunshine Products.*

Marti Wheeler, a natural hygienist and writer for the Health Excellence System, questions whether we should even drink eight glasses of water daily as recommended by nutritionists. It is claimed that water "flushes" out the body and keeps it clean. Wheeler claims this idea is totally false since the body is entirely self-cleansing.

We overwork our bodies if we consume water beyond the demands of thirst. Most thirst results from improper eating habits, such as using salt, or spices which are toxic and irritating and must be held in solution until they are eliminated. In addition, soy sauces, miso, dulse, kelp, and seaweeds are high in inorganic salt and cause great thirst.

Cooking deranges the nutrients in foods, and these deranged nutrients are toxic, causing thirst. Like seasonings, deranged nutrients must be held in solution until they can be eliminated.

Wheeler concludes that uncooked fruits and vegetables, along with up to four ounces of raw nuts or seeds daily, provide all the nutrients and pure water you need without causing pathological thirst. Humans are not naturally water-drinking animals. The only time you may experience thirst when you're eating properly is during periods of fasting, rigorous activity, or exposure to heat.[25i]

ORAL CONTRACEPTIVE PILLS

Medical research indicates that oral contraceptive pills for women may lead to tinnitus, vertigo, and hearing loss.[12, p67]

Mindell lists the possible side effects from taking oral contraceptive pills: cramps, loss of appetite, nausea, acne, swelling of ankles and feet, tenderness and swelling of breasts, fatigue, diarrhea, skin rash, vaginal discharge, and increased blood pressure. If you smoke, the combination of estrogen and progesterone, makes you more susceptible to heart attacks, strokes, high blood pressure, and formation of hazardous blood clots in the veins.[40, pp114-116]

I list these seemingly unrelated symptoms because they all lead to using more drugs, which in turn lead to tinnitus.

Mindell adds that many Pill users are seriously deficient in folic acids, as well as vitamins C, E, and B-1, B-2, B-6, B-12, and essential minerals such as zinc and magnesium.

Mindell offers a reference list of foods that contain the vitamins and minerals mentioned.

POOR DIET

I repeat what Yanick said previously: The inner ear contains thousands of specialized sensory cells which need water, oxygen, and a suitable combination of about 40 nutrients all blended in the right proportions. All parts of the ear require nutrients in order to effectively deliver complete electrical information to the brain.[34]

The American Tinnitus Association holds that a healthy diet avoids the following foods, all high in sodium salts: ham, bacon, and processed meat such as bologna and frankfurters; fat from meat; duck and goose; canned, salted or smoked meat or fish; shellfish; cheese, except unsalted cottage cheese; canned baked beans and soup; pickles, olives, and prepared sauces; soft drinks and prepared beverage mixes; candy; baking powder and soda; and salted potato chips, popcorn, corn chips, pretzels, and peanuts.[7c]

Many of these foods become rancid during processing or by the time they reach your table.

Airola contends that rancid foods are harmful to the entire body. During the oxidation process leading to rancidity, harmful chemical substances are produced. In foods, these substances irritate the delicate linings of the stomach and intestines. Prolonged use of rancid oils and other foods can under some conditions, have a carcinogenic effect. Also, rancid oils destroy vitamins E, F (essential fatty acids), A, and carotene. Paavo Airola discusses rancidity at length in the book, You Are Confused?

Airola explains that whole wheat flour at room temperature turns rancid in just a few days. Most vegetable oils turn rancid in a matter of weeks, especially if kept in transparent glass containers at room temperature. Most unhulled or unshelled seeds and nuts with a high oil content turn rancid in less than a year. He points out that rancid fats and oils are used extensively in processing such foods as doughnuts, roasted nuts and seeds (actually not roasted but cooked in oil heated to an extremely high temperature), bakery foods, pies, potato chips, deep-fried restaurant foods, and commercially-fried chicken.[19a]

The Junk Food Withdrawal Manual, is an excellent book to help you improve your diet.[43]

PRESCRIPTION DRUGS

This section is aimed at "drug misuse." The negative effects of drugs on the hearing apparatus has already been established.

Some of man's earliest medicines were derived from natural plant products to ward off pain. One of those substances, morphine, a derivative from the opium poppy, remains one of the most powerful drugs we have for pain relief. Cocaine is a derivative of the coca leaf, and it has important medical use as a local anesthetic.

Natural and synthetic opiates make up the class of drugs known as the narcotic analgesics. An analgesic is a drug that kills pain without causing loss of consciousness. A narcotic is a type of drug that depresses the nervous system and produces effects similar to those of morphine, such as sedation and a pleasant state of euphoria.

The opiate narcotics have been a mixed blessing in the annals of medicine. Throughout history their remarkable analgesic effects have relieved the suffering of countless numbers of people. But there is a difference between "drug use", "drug misuse," and "drug abuse." The physical problems arise from the abuse and misuse of drugs. Drug use is the ingesting a drug for its intended purpose and in the appropriate dosage and frequency. Drug misuse is using a drug for its intended purpose but taking it in greater amounts. Drug abuse is the deliberate use of a drug for a reason other than its intended purpose and in doses that are potentially damaging to the user.

Opiates, analgesics and narcotics are used in antidiarrheals, tranquilizers, antihistamines, sedatives, antidepressants, muscle relaxants, anesthetics, cough suppressants, pain relievers, and pulmonary edemas (swelling of the lungs).

The following narcotics are found in prescription drugs: propoxyphene, meperidine, oxycodone, oxymorphone, levorphanol, hydrocodone, hydromorphone, pentazocine, butorphanol, or nalbuphine.[22c]

According to Fry, some 5 million Americans are so poisoned by medicines each year as to require hospitalization. And 200,000 die annually from Physician-administered drugs. He lists antipyrine, barbiturates, nitrobenzol, salvarsan...the list goes on and on.[25d]

John Oliver, a La Mesa, CA, pharmacist, wrote as follows in Emergency magazine:

"Drugs affect multiple systems of the body. No drug is specific for a particular target area in the body to the exclusion of any other physiological system...Drugs are taken too much for granted; they are not accorded the skepticism they deserve.

The human body is not designed to take drugs. Whenever a drug is introduced into the body, the defensive mechanisms immediately begin to protect the system by neutralizing or eliminating the invader. Drugs are poison. Why else would the body neutralize and eliminate them?

A drug will not cause the body to do anything it cannot, of itself, do. It will do one of two things: it will stimulate or (it will) depress a physiological function. It cannot create a new function."[25e]

Robert S. Mendelsohn, in his book, Confessions of a Medical Heretic says: "Don't trust your doctor. Assume that if he (sic) prescribes a drug, it's dangerous. There is no safe drug. Eli Lilly himself once said that a drug without toxic effects is no drug at all. Every drug has to be approached with suspicion."[44]

QUINIDINE

Black's Medical Dictionary defines quinidine as an alkaloid that is closely related to the chemical composition and the action to quinidine. It is used in the treatment of the cardiac irregularity known as atrial fibrillation.[45]

Isadore Rosenfeld, MD, in his book, Modern Prevention: The New Medicine tells of a heart patient who was given quinidine, causing tinnitus so loud that she thought there was construction going on outside her window. The drug was stopped immediately, and her symptoms cleared up. Rosenfeld listed quinidine along with many other drugs that can cause deafness. He stated that drug-induced deafness is insidious, progressive, often unrecognized and occasionally permanent.[46]

Airola contends that the basic cause of heart disease can be found in faulty eating and living habits and various mental and physical environment stresses. The following are major risk factors in coronary heart disease. Note that most of them are of dietary origin:

a. Elevated blood levels of cholesterol, triglycerides, and other fatty substances.
b. Elevated blood pressure.
c. Elevated blood uric acid levels (mainly caused by high protein diet).
d. Certain metabolic disorders, notably diabetes.
e. Obesity.
f. Smoking.
g. Lack of physical exercise.

Airola suggests a lacto-vegetarian, low-sodium, low-calorie, low-animal-protein diet of high quality, featuring natural foods with emphasis on whole grains, seeds and nuts, fresh fruits and vegetables.

Airola lists the following foods and supplements as beneficial in a heart condition. Buckwheat is rich in rutin, which keeps arteries in good health. Bananas and potatoes are rich in potassium, which is vital for healthy heart function. Okra helps reduce blood vessel friction. Apples contain pectin, which is of great benefit in atherosclerosis. Flax seed oil is rich in essential fatty acids, especially in linoleic acid. Asparagus is beneficial for an enlarged heart.

Airola cautions against salt, sugar, alcohol, coffee, meat, processed foods, animal and processed fats (margarine). Don't overeat. Don't smoke. Don't drink chlorinated water, which destroys vitamin E in the body. Avoid smog, and emotional stresses, and worries.[19, pp101-104]

QUININE

Quinine and other antimalarial drugs have long been known for their ability to produce temporary hearing loss and tinnitus. Quinine-induced hearing loss and tinnitus are apparently of high frequency, and the tinnitus onset reportedly precedes the hearing loss. Some reports indicate that in sensitive individuals the quinine contained in a single gin-and-tonic highball can be adequate to produce tinnitus.[47]

Quinine produces irreversible nerve hearing loss, which also may be transmitted from a pregnant woman to her fetus.[24, p288]

Black states that quinine hydrochloride has been used with urethane as a sclerosing agent in the treatment of varicose veins. Quinine is used as an antipyretic for combating fevers.[45] But medical views on suppressing fevers is changing. An article by Jane E. Brody, a science writer for the New York Times, reported that many of today's doctors are re-evaluating their view on suppressing fevers and are allowing them to run their course, since studies show that fevers may shorten illness and reduce the chances of spreading infection to others. Fevers reportedly mobilize the body's immunological defenses against infectious organisms and, in some cases, directly inhibit their growth.

The article goes on to say that high fevers are not safe for some people, since fever imposes a high energy

51

cost on the individual. For each 1-degree Celsius rise in body temperature, the body's metabolic rate increases about 10 percent. This means that heart rate, respiration, and other metabolic functions are speeded up. The elderly, people with heart disease, newborn infants, and others may suffer undue stress from fevers, especially prolonged ones.[48]

SALICYLATE

Salicylate is the active ingredient of aspirin, taken often by many people to relieve headaches and other aches and pains.

Aspirin, or course, is the most commonly used drug known for its effects on hearing and tinnitus. After just 48 hours on a dosage of about 4.8 grams a day, there is 10-15 dB of hearing loss, and this can grow with continued use to as much as 40-50 dB. Upon termination of the drug, the hearing loss almost always recovers within 24-72 hours, depending upon the serum salicylate level achieved.[36, p60]

Rodale remarks that aspirin is an irritant to the stomach lining. Taking aspirin for rheumatic pains over a long period of time may cause any or all of the following: nausea, heartburn, stomach pain, deafness, dizziness, ringing in the ears. Doctors generally wait for their arthritic patients who are taking aspirin to tell them that their ears are ringing before they prescribe a cut in dosage. That is the sign that the patient has overdosed.[6, p347]

Many headaches are a symptom of ingesting foods that you are allergic to, and which are swallowed too quickly (see Allergies). Breathing perfume, or toxic odors, or stress can bring on a headache.editor

As an alternative to aspirin for pain reduction, Mindell recommends 100 milligrams of niacin, 3 times daily, and 100 milligrams of stress B complex (time release), twice daily. Calcium and magnesium (twice as much calcium as magnesium is the proper ratio), which are nature's tranquilizers.[18, p182]

Using aspirin for the pain of arthritis eliminates only the symptom and does not cure arthritis. Depending on the level to which your physical condition has deteriorated, a proper diet may reverse it. Several of my friends have been helped by the following books:

There Is a Cure for Arthritis, by Paavlo Airola[19]

I Cured My Arthritis: You Can Too, by Margie Garrison[49]

Aspirin is also used for migraine headaches. Doctors Herbert M. Shelton and William L. Esser state that the more migraine sufferers are drugged to relieve their headaches, the more toxic their body's become. The very treatments employed to help, instead perpetuate and intensify the suffering.

The discomfort associated with migraine headaches is actually the body in the process of attempting to eliminate the build-up of toxins, which developed from improper foods, drugs and stress. Nature is trying to force the body to rest to prevent the accumulation of more toxins.

Shelton and Esser suggest a period of fasting with

complete rest, away from all immediate troubles. The fasting should occur under the direct supervision of one who understands this method of treatment.[25f]

Natural Hygienists have knowledge of supervising fasts. A list of Natural Hygiene Retreats is given under Resources.

SUGAR

Lamb states that the fatty-cholesterol deposits that occur in arteries (atherosclerosis) obstruct the circulation to the ear.[3, p2]

John Yudkin, MD, states in his book <u>Sweet and Dangerous</u> that sugar is a major contributing factor in atherosclerosis.[50]

Bidwell stated in her article "Objections to the Standard American Diet" that refined sugars cause depletion of vital alkaline minerals. The body must then "borrow" precious alkaline minerals from teeth and bones to metabolize demineralized white sugar. (editor: That includes the bones in the ear.)

Refined sugar, Bidwell continues, contributes to blood sugar disorders. A half pound of apples contains 132 calories, whereas a half pound of candy has 900. This is concentrated sugar far beyond what the human body was ever adapted to deal with at one sitting.

Furthermore, refined sugar contributes to heart disease. Large doses of sugar cause the insulin to convert blood glucose (sugar) into fatty acids and triglycerides (blood fat). People on a high-sugar diet develop significantly high levels of blood fat. The high triglycerides are directly related to development of hardening of the arteries.

Finally, Bidwell states, sugar is a major contributor to tooth decay and gum disease, obesity, diabetes, hypertension and heart disease, hypoglycemia, vitamin deficiencies, and psychological disorders.[25g]

E. M. Abrahamson, MD, and A. W. Pezet add to the list of illnesses in their book Body, Mind, & Sugar. Sugar aggravates tendencies toward diverticulosis, colon cancer, and osteoporosis, and it "feeds" fungi such as Candida albicans.[51]

Along with these illnesses goes a plethora of "curative" medicines and drugs many of which aggravate tinnitus.

Yudkin asserted that there is no physiological requirement for sugar. All human nutritional needs and the avidity for sweetness can be met in full by eating natural foods. Sugar is the only "food" that supplies nothing whatsoever in the way of nutrients.[50, p3]

The consumption of sugar on top of an ordinary diet increases the risk of obesity. Nutritional deficiencies develop with the consumption of sugar. Yudkin backs up Bidwell's statement about heart disease by telling of a 1957 report by a Japanese researcher confirming the relationship between sugar intake and coronary heart disease in twenty countries.[pp50, 30, 92]

All foods with artificial sweeteners or sugar should be slowly eliminated from your diet. Begin by replacing after-dinner snacks with fruit. (Wait at least 45 minutes to 1 hour after a protein meal before eating fruit which digests in the intestinal tract and not the stomach, otherwise you will suffer from indigestion.) And because sugar is a drug, you will suffer withdrawal symptoms. Give your body time to acclimate itself to the change in diet.[editor]

I eliminated sugar from my diet 20 years ago by slowly deleting those foods that required sugar. I read in Prevention magazine about eating a dill pickle when there was a craving for sweets. I tried it and the craving disappeared! Of course, pickles are packed with preservatives, but snacking on them is a temporary measure until you lose your craving for sweets. Sugar is more detrimental to the body than the preservatives.

Below are two books that explain the detrimental effects of sugar on the entire body:

Sugar Blues[52]
Natural Health, Sugar and the
Criminal Mind[53]

TRANQUILIZERS

Usoa Busto, MD, writing for the New England Journal of Medicine states that tranquilizers such as Valium, Dalmane, Librium, and Ativan may cause tinnitus when stopped after the drugs are used for several years. The ringing generally disappears within four or five weeks and is less severe if the user gradually reduces dosage rather than stops "cold turkey." We in the self-help group, have found that once the ringing starts, quitting and then restarting the tranquilizers will prolong the tinnitus.[54]

I share the following experience with you even though I now realize I made a foolish choice. In attempting to end my dependency on Ativan (a sleeping pill I used some time ago), I took my doctor's advice about trying an over-the-counter remedy named Unisom Dual Relief, produced by Pfizer. After the very first dose I suffered three days of horrible side effects: drowsiness, a feeling of heaviness in my chest, and general weakness. On the positive side, however, the tinnitus quieted to barely a whisper for about five days. My doctor had said the drug might quiet down my tinnitus. He was right about that.

If you should use Unisom, let me know the results. Take note of the warning label which states that people suffering from asthma, arthritis, glaucoma, and enlarged prostate should use the product only under the advice and supervision of a physician. And yet this is an FDA-approved product.

There are less intrusive aids for withdrawing from tranquilizers. Many bookstores have an excellent selection of books that guide you in techniques of mental relaxation. I find relaxation tape cassettes very helpful. I can listen to them while doing other things and while going to sleep. Excellent tapes may be obtained from:

Potentials Unlimited, Inc.*

I recommend the tape Astral Sounds because it has helped me. It is a unique hour-long cassette produced by the American Research Team, available from Potentials Unlimited. Instead of containing human voices, musical instruments, or sounds of the environment such as rain, wind, or the ocean, it plays very delicate sound waves generated from a computer program created by a team of psychologists. The sound waves and sound frequencies are arranged in a specific pattern claimed to have profound positive psychological effects on the mind and body of the listener.

Acquaintances who have used this tape report that it removes physical pain, cures insomnia, reduces stress and anxiety, provides instant and deep relaxation, makes them happy and naturally high, and creates magnificent visual imagery. And all without drugs!

If you are dependent on tranquilizers to help you sleep, Traditional Medicinals produces an herb tea named "Nighty Night,"* which is very effective. Most grocery stores now carry their products.

After drinking a calming herb tea and going to bed, try the following visualization exercise. It is more effective than physical exercise for me.

Imagine the following: clasp your hands together, bend your elbows, then touch each knee with the opposite elbow (right elbow to left knee, left elbow to right knee), while you say "Ohm." Keep repeating the exercise. Don't stop. Sleep will come soon.

If books, teas, and tapes are not effective, consider questioning your life-style. If you feel that your way of life is driving you to dependency on tranquilizers, wouldn't it be better for your physical and mental health simply to change it? When your physical condition gets so desperate, all the money and doctors in the world will be unable to help you regain your health. Tranquilizers cause a chemical imbalance in the body that eventually causes organ dysfunction. Peace of mind and body are more important than money, position, and impressing people. Recall the steps you made while you were advancing to the economic and social position you are in. At what level-with what life-style-where you most comfortable?

Perhaps the following quote will be helpful. "We spend the first half of our lives gaining wealth at the expense of our health, and the second half of our lives spending our wealth to regain our health." (Author unknown to me.)

The section on "Nicotine" gives further suggestions on how to break an addiction.

DENTAL FLOSS

Hulda Regehr Clark, Ph.D., N.D., explains in her book Cure For All Cancers*, not to use dental floss because the floss has been coated with mercury antiseptics. The mercury will enter your blood stream in seconds, and travel to the ear canal. Clark recommends using 2-pound monofilament fish line. Also, throw away all of your old toothbrushes, because they are contaminated from the mercury.

*Under BOOKS in RESOURCE section.

CHEMICALS

ANILINE

Aniline is used in the manufacture of hair dyes, medicinals, resins, and perfumes. Intoxication may occur from inhalation, ingestion, or absorption through the skin. Serious poisoning from ingestion causes acute lack of oxygen in the blood, dizziness, headache, mental confusion, and skin lesions. Tumors have been reported in animals whose skins were painted with coal-tar dye. Aniline is also called phenylamine.[29, p31]

Hair dyes of all kinds are strongly advised against if there is any head noise. These substances definitely affect the hearing adversely, and although it is again difficult to determine whether this is a direct or indirect result, experience proves that their use is detrimental to the scalp and arterial and nervous systems. Many women who continually dye their hair gradually have trouble with headaches, skin ailments, hearing difficulties and head noises. This is because the scalp is frequently used by the body as an eliminative tissue, and it is most effective if kept clean, washed regularly and brushed in the ordinary way.

The cleansing powers of the body are much reduced by the use of hair dyes, with the result that the impurities which were being pushed through the scalp then become submerged in the lower or innermost layers and affect the brain tissues and the apparatus of hearing. There is no actual benefit in undergoing any treatment if the hair is going to be continually dyed. There would be an appreciable relief immediately when dyeing is stopped and replaced only by general hair hygiene.

Again it must be understood tht many sweets contain dyes and chemicals which can affect the nervous system and may cause head noises. These must be stopped, and whenever possible the sugar in the diet should be obtained from honey and the other natural sweet foods.[55, p63]

Stay away from resins and varnishes. There are no present alternatives to these chemicals.[editor]

ARSENIC

This poison and its compounds are found in hair tonics and hair dyes (which can cause contact dermatitis), fungicides, pesticides, dyes, paints, artists' colors, veterinary drugs, and cigarette smoke. In medical use it's employed to treat spirochetal infections, blood disorders, and skin diseases. Chronic poisoning can result in pigmentation of skin and liver, and liver damage.[29, p34]

Some homeopathic remedies also contain arsenic, labeled as arsenium. Read the labels before you use these products.[editor]

ARTIFICIAL FLAVORINGS

Artificial flavorings are technology's counterfeit food, writes Vickey Bidwell in her article, "Objections to Synthetic Food." One example: A flavoring product is labeled "Imitation Strawberry." Its ingredients list: vanilla and other aldehydes, ethyl butyrate and other esters, oil of lemon and other essential oils, Butyric and other acids, benzodihydropone, iodine and other ketones, alcohol, propylene glycol, water, artificial color, and 0.1% benzoate of soda.[25g]

Our digestive system is not biologically adapted to assimilate these chemicals, thus they become entrenched in the tissues.

Toxins can leave the body cells only through the elimination system, through perspiration from physical activity, or through fasting. Artificial flavors can be replaced with fresh fruits.[25h]

BENZENE

Benzene is a solvent derived from coal and used in nail polish remover. It is also found in varnishes, airplane dopes, lacquers, and as a solvent for waxes, resins and oils. Harmful amounts may be absorbed through the skin.[29, p4]

This chemical is also used in weed killers, glues, detergents, aspirin, insecticides, analgesic drugs, fabric dyes, and dry-cleaning solvents. Chromosome damage and birth defects in rats have been attributed to it.

Although additional research is indicated,

benzene has been implicated as a causative factor in marrow atrophy and some forms of leukemia. Benzene also has been identified as a cause of defective development of tissues.[56]

An alternative to benzene for spot cleaning is baking soda. Sprinkle it on, brush it in, then vacuum it off. Test this treatment on an unnoticeable area first, as it tends to lighten fabric.[editor]

Dry cleaners use such chemicals as ammonia, benzene, chlorine, formaldehyde, glycerin, naphthalene, paraffin, perchloroethylene, toluene, trichloroethylene, and xylene. Always remove garments from their polyethylene wrapping outside when you get them home and air them out in the fresh air before you wear them.[16, pp92-93]

Find a cleaner who will use naphtha as the solvent instead of perchorethane derivative; it seems to be less odoriferous and is often tolerated by those with chemical sensitivities.[editor]

FOOD PRESERVATIVES AND ADDITIVES

Saifer and Zellerback submit the following points in their book, Detox:

The FDA defines a food additive as "any substance that becomes part of a food product when added either directly or indirectly." Today, more than 3,890 chemicals are intentionally added to produce desired effects; 10,000 other compounds find their way into foods during processing and storage. It is estimated that the average American ingests one gallon of food additives yearly.

Because additives tend to be present in much larger quantities than pesticides they cause more general toxicity. Many on the FDA's "Generally Recognized as Safe" list have not been adequately tested for harmful effects on humans.

Not all additives are harmful or toxic. When fresh food is unattainable, preservatives delay spoilage and ensure that we will not suffer hunger. Many commercial products are fortified with vitamins and minerals (often to replace those lost in processing). And "safe" or "natural" ingredients such as lecithin, an emulsifier, can sometimes improve texture and flavor.

There is much dispute about the harmful effects a steady diet of these chemicals can cause. Occasional small exposures to any one additive should not cause problems, but the long-term effect of daily exposures to a variety of additives has not been laboratory tested. Some persons "miraculously" recover from "incurable" ailments such as arthritis or schizophrenia three or four days after they change to a diet of unprocessed foods.[23, pp42-43]

LEAD, HYDROCARBONS, CARBON MONOXIDE

Gasoline service attendants are particularly susceptible to these poisons, which are present in both unburned gasoline and tailpipe emissions. Gasoline fumes at the pump are a major source of exposure for most people.[6, p32]

If you are sensitive to the fumes (do you notice a tinnitus flare-up after you have filled your tank?), ask someone else to fill it for you or go to a full-service station and keep the windows rolled up. It's worth the extra pennies not to aggravate the tinnitus. Many states require fume emission controls on the filling nozzle, and lead compounds are gradually being phased out as gasoline antiknock additives.

Lead oxide is also being phased out as a component in paint, but it is unfortunate that reports are still heard of toddlers being poisoned from chewing on old painted surfaces.[editor]

A report by Arnold R. Saslow, MD and Paul S. Clark, MD, in the Journal of Occupational Medicine, tells of an outbreak of carbon monoxide poisoning involving a natural gas heater malfunctioning at a sports arena in Alaska. Those who were affected by the carbon monoxide complained of headaches, dizziness, nausea, tinnitus, disorientation, and numbness of extremities.[57]

NATURAL AND BOTTLED GAS

Small amounts of gas used for cooking and heating can seep from the supply lines or burners. The gas company inserts a characteristic odor into the gas to make any leaks noticeable. Have the supplier check the lines if anyone detects even the slightest odor.[editor]

MERCURY

Since July of 1973, all mercury which was widely used in cosmetics was banned by the FDA except as a preservative in eye preparations to inhibit the growth of germs. It may cause a variety of symptoms ranging from chronic inflammation of the mouth and gums to personality changes, nervousness, fever, rash and if ingested in small amounts it may be fatal.[29, p143]

I mention the above symptoms and dangers because the FDA still allows mercury amalgams to be used as dental fillings.

The antiamalgamists are basing their renewed push on two recent studies conducted in Canada, and discussed in a recent Insight magazine article. One study, led by Dr. Murray J. Vimy, suggests that mercury leaves the amalgams and accumulates in tissues and that brushing teeth or chewing gum can exert enough pressure to transform the solid amalgam into a vapor that can be swallowed.

In the article, Dr. Fritz Lorscheider, states: "Mercury is highly permeable to cell membranes and as a vapor can readily move across the lungs to the blood and to the gastrointestinal tract...Once mercury is in the blood, it can travel to other organs."[58]

Poisoning from silver-mercury amalgam has been increasing at an alarming rate since it was first introduced in the United States in 1825, according to Hal A. Huggins, DDS., author of It's All In Your Head. Huggins has made a study of the effects of silver-mercury fillings on our general health. He recently took a poll of 1,320 of his patients and found that almost half of them complained of constant or frequent ringing or noise in their ears. The list of 30 symptoms is available from Dr. Huggins on request.

For tinnitus sufferers, the removal of silver-mercury fillings may help, but they must be removed in quadrants and in a certain order to keep your general condition from worsening. Huggins explains the procedure in his book. He can also be reached by phone at 1-800-331-2303.

Huggins also has a referral list of dentists around the country familiar with determining mercury toxicity in patients and sequential removal of this offending metal from the teeth.[59]

Joyal Taylor, DDS, makes some interesting comments in his book, Mercury Toxicity From Dental Fillings. Proteins are important for hormone and enzyme production cell growth and repair, genetics, and the manufacture of antibodies. Mercury may cause an imbalance of protein in the body, inactivate sulfhydryl bonds found in some amino acids, and affect the protein of white blood cells that are responsible for many immune responses. It is also capable of adversely affecting the protein components in cell replication by altering DNA molecules.

Insufficient protein can affect the immune system, as well as imbalance the body chemistry in general, due to its importance in the endocrine system, glands, and hormones. Overcooking and micro waving of meats cause the protein in them to become inactive. Drinking liquids with meals disturbs protein digestion.

Mercury-toxified patients may show improvement in protein metabolism with proper dietary protein intake, digestive enzymes, and free form amino acid supplements if properly combined with silver mercury filling removal.[60]

Taylor offers suggestions on finding a qualified

dentist to remove mercury fillings.[60, p115] I have listed most of the organizations under REFERENCES that Taylor lists in his book to help you find dentists who believe mercury fillings should be removed.

I have also listed the address and phone number of a dentist in Tijuana, Mexico, Joaquin Zavala C, DDS. I know two people who had their fillings removed by Zavala, and were very happy with his service.

A nutritional supplement which assists in detoxification and in the chelation of trace amounts of heavy metals is TOXSANS. It is available from Arizona Natural Products, listed under "HERBS" in RESOURCES.

SULFUR

This element is used in matches, medicine, gunpowder, and vulcanized rubber. In place of matches, liquid-fueled, or gas-fueled lighters, the sensitive person can purchase a piezoelectric lighter from camping supply stores. It is hand-held and looks like a giant safety pin. Squeezing it causes a heating element to glow to ignition temperatures, like the electric cigarette lighter in a car.

Also people who are sensitive to sulfur dioxide should avoid fruit and raisins preserved other than by sun or vacuum drying. Most wines have a low level of sulfur compounds, some more than others.[editor]

69

PHYSICAL CAUSES

DIVING

C. Edmonds wrote an article titled "Hearing Loss With Frequent Diving (deaf divers) in Undersea Biomedical Research. The presence of permanent hearing loss and its associated tinnitus in caisson (a large watertight chamber within which work is done underwater, as on a bridge pier) workers has long been established. In 1913 a doctor coined the phrase, "caisson worker's deafness" to describe a hearing loss which was either acute or chronic, temporary or permanent. A 1971 study of caisson workers under 40 years of age found that 60 percent had hearing defects.

Other factors controlling why caisson workers are affected with a high incidence of hearing abnormalities, include atmospheric pressure, decompression sickness, infections, and noise damage.

Despite the current acceptance of the disorder of permanent hearing loss as an occupational complication of diving, there is very little evidence of the incidence of this disorder among skin divers.[61]

FLYING

The American Tinnitus Association recommends several precautionary measures concerning flying. Don't fly if you have a cold because, particularly during descent from altitude, the eardrum is subjected to rapid pressure change. If the eustachian tube is plugged from the inflammation and swelling of a cold, it can't equalize air pressure on either side of the eardrum fast enough to cope with this change, and aerotitis (traumatic inflammation of the middle ear) can result. Serious inner-ear trauma may occur when a fistula (a duct formed by the imperfect closing of an abscess) develops in the oval or round windows of the fragile inner ear structure. Endolymphatic fluid (the fluid filling the membranous labyrinth of the ear) leaks out, causing hearing loss and dizziness. Rupture of the inner-ear membranes can result in total hearing loss.

If you must fly when you have a cold, here are a few tips that will lessen the possibility of acquiring tinnitus. Use ear plugs during ascent and descent, and after landing leave them in long enough for the eardrum pressure to equalize, perhaps until you reach the main terminal. Other tips are to chew gum, to yawn, and to pinch your nose and blow gently. Also use nasal decongestants one-half hour before descent.[7b]

A small device is available to relieve ear pain when flying. It was developed by a physician after he experienced ear discomfort during an airplane flight. The device is a small, compact, sturdy plastic container, which is filled with warm water and placed over the ear. The heat travels to the middle ear and relieves pressure caused by changes in altitude and cabin pressure. Pain and discomfort are lessened within minutes. The product's name is *Ear Ease* and is available from Norm Thompson.* It is listed under HEARING PRODUCTS.

HEAD BLOWS

Traumas to the head have been shown to cause serious high frequency hearing loss. Physical shocks experienced in contact sports such as football, rugby, wrestling, and in particular boxing can cause hearing loss. Since the damage normally affects only the higher range of frequencies, it is usually the "quality" of speech that is affected; because quality is so subjective, this damage often goes undetected for years.[12, p57]

HIGH-IMPACT AEROBICS

A recent report in the New England Journal of Medicine, by Michael A. Weintraub, MD, warns that physical exercises that lift both feet off the ground at once may damage the hearing. The repeated jarring of the body as the feet impact a hard surface apparently can disturb delicate parts of the inner ear and cause imbalance, vertigo, tinnitus and hearing loss.

Weintraub explains that the continuous bouncing up and down causes vibrations to be transmitted to the skull and tiny bones of the inner ear. When the otoliths in the inner ear are dislodged, it's irreversible. Despite the routine use of special cushioned shoes to enhance shock absorption, injuries occur.[62]

I only jump on my rebounder (a miniature trampoline), and only for five minutes. Any time longer than that will cause my tinnitus to flare up.

LOOSE HAIRS IN EAR CANAL

George Goldman of Massachusetts Institute of Technology (MIT) has treated several patients complaining of tinnitus who have had an ear hair floating close to the eardrum. When the loose hair vibrates, it causes an unusually loud noise similar to "distant thunder." You can attempt to remove the hair yourself by using a syringe, and rinsing the ear. If that is not successful, a doctor can remove it by using forceps.[63]

WHIPLASH INJURY AND HEAD TRAUMA

J. U. Toglia reported in the Journal of Forensic Sciences, that complaints concerning faulty inner ear functions are common following whiplash or other head injuries. Such complaints include vertigo, "unsteadiness," tinnitus, hearing loss, and difficulty in understanding speech. Records kept on 72 patients who had whiplash injury and head trauma, show that 37 complained of tinnitus who never experienced such sounds before.[64]

INTERNAL CAUSATIVE DISORDERS

ALLERGIES

McFadden remarked that it is believable that any allergic reaction directly or indirectly affects the three parts of the ear: outer, middle, or inner systems could also be accompanied by tinnitus. For example, any food or inhalant allergy that caused a blockage of the Eustachian tube might produce tinnitus as a by-product. Diet plays a very important role in tinnitus management. Coffee, tea, tonic water, red wine, grain-based spirits, cheese, and chocolate have been the most common dietary causes of tinnitus.[36, p81]

Soraya Hoover, MD, of Houston, Texas, analyzed 75 tinnitus patients by using blood tests, Ct scans, x-rays, a tinnitus synthesizer, audiological equipment, and allergy tests. The following chart, from an American Tinnitus Association Newsletter report of Hoover's study, shows the percentage of the total number of subjects in whom various foods and other factors induced short-term tinnitus.[7d]

Foods, other factors	Percentage of subjects affected
Dairy Products	****************18
Pork	***********11
Wheat	*********9
Coffee	********8
Chicken	******6
Chocolate.	*****5
Corn	*****5
Eggs	*****5
Beef	****4
Potatoes	****4
Smoking	****4
Tomatoes	***3
Alcohol	**2
Broccoli	**2
Garlic	**2
Outdoor pollens	**2
Pinto Beans	**2
Rice	**2
Apples	*1
Bell Peppers	*1
Onions	*1
Oranges	*1
Peanuts	*1
Tea	*1

(Editor's note: Could the reaction to the fresh fruits and vegetables on the list be due to residual pesticides?)

For information about allergy self-testing, see the ADDENDUM at the end of this book. For more information about these studies of the relationship between allergies and tinnitus, write:

Soraya Hoover, MD*

The American Medical Association Encyclopedia defines allergy as a collection of disease symptoms caused by exposure of the skin to a chemical, of the respiratory system to particles of dust or pollen, or of the stomach and intestines to a particular food, which in the majority of people causes no symptoms.

The function of the immune system is to recognize antigens (foreign proteins), and to form antibodies and sensitized white blood cells that will interact with these antigens, leading to their destruction.[65]

Chester P. Yozwick presents it differently. He quotes Herbert M. Shelton, MD: "Allergy is a specific lack of body tolerance to a long-term toxemic condition. This condition is the basic cause of all inflammations of the lining membranes of the hollow organs of the body."

So long as overindulgence in denatured food is continued, it is impossible to overcome allergies. "Allergies" as well as tooth decay, pimples, headaches, flu, colds, diabetes, heart trouble, cancer, arthritis, etc., are not causes, but symptoms, of the overall condition of the body. Any of these symptoms mark the end point of the body's tolerance for accumulation of internal waste matter. The body, in this condition, usually has an acid excess and an alkali depletion.

The answer lies in detoxification by fasting and proper modes of living, such as maintaining a proper acid-alkali balance through proper diet, exercise, pure water, ample rest, sunshine, and fresh air.[25j]

Fry dispels the theory of "allergies," and claims that only healthy people have a vital resistance to reject toxins in food. Some of the foods that contain toxins are

77

wheat, eggs, milk, chocolate and nuts. Wheat contains gluten and phytic acid which beget toxic conditions in the eater because humans don't have the enzymes to deal with these two components. Beans have anti-enzyme factors that make them indigestible in their raw state. Chocolate contains theobromine,a poisonous cousin of caffeine. Milk contains casein and lactose, which people over the age of three lack the enzymes to digest. And nuts, like beans, protect themselves with tannic acid, prussic acid (as in almond skins), and anti-enzyme factors.[25k]

Nature has provided early mother's milk with colostrum, explains Fry, an ingredient that helps develop the baby's immune system as an aid in fighting infections and allergies prior to development of its own immune system. Most allergies are the result of feeding babies such foods as cereals, meat, and whole cow's milk before the age of 10 to 12 months. Until then, babies do not secrete the salivary enzyme, ptyalin, the pancreatic and intestinal enzymes essential to digestion of adult foods. Nature tells us when babies are ready for solid foods: their teeth develop, permitting them to chew.[25 l]

Babies who are fed starch foods too early suffer from indigestion, colic, diarrhea, constipation, colds, hives, and tonsillar and adenoidal troubles. Allergic reactions to starches in infancy carry into adulthood.[25m]

For more information on nutrition and motherhood, write to:

Health Excellence Systems*

Ask for The Health Reporter, Volume 1, No. 9. The 1990 price is $3.50, plus $2.50 shipping.

In a subsequent issue of The Health Reporter, Fry writes: "Allergies are believed to be a problem of over-sensitization from a desperate body that has lost its normal bearing. The body has become irrational in its response to substances."

The problem is quickly solved by removing the causes of the over-sensitization, usually the underlying toxins, by discontinuing all except the most basic activities. Even food can be dispensed with. Under the condition of a fast, the body can redirect all available energies to cleansing and normalization. One to two weeks of fasting is usually sufficient to overcome the problem.[25n]

After you have gone through this cleansing process, start on a rotation diet, which means not eating any particular food more than once every five days until you discover what foods you are allergic to. Eliminate that food from your diet for six to eight weeks, then try it again for verification. For more information on the rotation diet, the book, 5-Day Allergy Relief System, by Marshall Mandell, MD, is available in health food stores.

In his book Mandell writes that to isolate the particular allergens responsible for an individual's reactions, clinical ecologists suggest a 10-day to 2-month elimination of the following most highly allergenic foods: eggs, wheat, white potatoes, all milk products, and oranges. He adds that a juice diet (many people call it a juice fast, but only the drinking of water is a true fast[editor]), is the most efficient way to eliminate allergies.[66]

Fasting (discussed in more detail in a later section of this book), is a highly individual matter, and I suggest that you study the practice in depth before engaging in it. If you are overweight by more than 50 pounds, seek the advice of a physician, naturopath, or natural hygienist. Natural hygienists are usually not listed separately in the phone book. Many chiropractors are also natural hygienists. A list of natural hygienists are in the RESOURCE section.

An audio cassette designed to eliminate allergies is available. Its producers believe that if you can change your mind, you can change your body. Tape 043, "Freedom from Allergies," is available from

Potentials Unlimited, Inc.*

ANEMIA

Rodale states that pernicious anemia can produce a soft ringing tinnitus. Symptoms of pernicious anemia are inflamed tongue, neuritis, degeneration of the spinal cord, upset stomach, extreme paleness, shortness of breath, and fatigue. The pernicious anemia patient lacks coordination of muscles, sways when standing with the eyes closed, loses a sense of position, and may have spasms.

The corrective diet should be predominantly alkaline, with emphasis on fruits and vegetables rich in iron: spinach, alfalfa, green onions, kale, broccoli, chard, okra, squash, carrots, beets, yams, tomatoes, bananas, red grapes, blueberries, black currants, prunes, and apricot juice. Other iron-rich foods are sunflower seeds, sesame seeds, peas and egg yolks.

Avoid tea and coffee because the caffeine in them interferes with iron absorption in the body.

Organic iron supplements are not recommended; the liver sources from which they are derived today are neither healthful nor nontoxic. Recommended supplements include vitamin B-12, B-6, pantothenic acid, B-complex, folic acid, PABA, vitamin E, betaine hydrochloride, and vitamin C.[6, p31 and pp809-811]

ANEURYSM

An aneurysm is the ballooning of an artery due to the pressure of blood flowing through a weakened area. The weakening may be due to disease, injury, or a congenital defect in the artery wall.[65, p113]

Lamb notes that an aneurysm is a rare cause of sounds from blood circulation in an artery or vein near the ear. This can be a nearly continuous sound, which increases in intensity as the blood is pumped out of the heart, and diminishes while the heart is relaxing and filling for the next beat. An x-ray to visualize the arteries and veins in the head is necessary to localize the problems. Usually this can be surgically corrected.[3, p3]

The symptoms of enlargement and bursting of a cerebral aneurysm is paralysis of eye movement, drooping of the lid, dilation of the pupil, neck rigidity, severe headache, and unconsciousness (symptoms similar to a stroke).[67, p113]

BRAIN TUMOR

Lamb submits that tinnitus can be the first sign of a brain tumor, but this is uncommon. A subjective, usually continuous low or high-pitched noise may be caused by a small tumor near the ear, in the brain area where the auditory nerve originates.[3, p3]

K. Thomsen, MD, et al, observed that when the tumor affects the region of the middle ear there will most often be hearing impairment and tinnitus as well as facial palsy. The tinnitus is usually the pulsating type.

This same report tells of 21 patients with tumors who were treated using surgery or irradiation, and the results of those treatments.[67]

Obviously, because of the possibility of a brain tumor, everyone who has tinnitus should get a thorough examination.[editor]

DIABETES

Bob Poppy, a science writer for Esquire magazine, has written an article about tinnitus titled, "What's the Buzz?" In it he makes the following statement, "Besides physical trauma, the causes of tinnitus include infections, diseases that restrict blood vessels thereby the hair cells' supply of nutrients (high cholesterol, high blood pressure, diabetes), and chemicals."[68]

Shelton explains that diabetes mellitus is the name given to a group of symptoms that center around an impairment of carbohydrate metabolism. Commonly we are told that it is a disease of the pancreas, but it is becoming clear that it is a disturbance of the metabolic process involving the entire organism and not strictly localized in any one organ.

The pancreas produces an internal secretion

commonly known as insulin which is essential to the oxidation of sugar. When it fails to secrete sufficient insulin, an excess sugar accumulates in the blood and is eliminated by the kidneys and urine. Hence sugar in the urine is the principal symptom of what the layman calls sugar diabetes.

There is no destruction in the pancreas when the disease first begins, and the destructive changes take place slowly against the weakened resistance of the body. Enervation (fatigue) of the tiny organs in the pancreas is probably the beginning of diabetes. It is toxemia that produces the pathology (destruction) in the pancreas.

Diabetes is on the increase in countries in which sugar consumption has grown rapidly the past 50 years—France, Germany, Britain and the United States. Every overweight person is a potential diabetic. The overfeeding which is responsible for the fat overworks the pancreas, and, as overwork of any organ results in impairment of the function of the organ, pancreatic failure result.

Excess carbohydrate places a strong stress on the pancreas. When this gland is overworked by too great an intake of starches and sugars, there first will be irritation and inflammation, then enlargement, followed by degeneration (de-secretion). After this, the body loses control of sugar metabolism, and an excess acidity is caused by too much starch and sugar.

But it should not be thought that overeating carbohydrates alone impairs the pancreas. Anything that produces enervation—tobacco, tea, coffee, chocolate, cocoa, alcohol, soda pop, sexual excesses, loss of sleep, overwork, general overeating, emotionalism, etc.—impairs organic function in general including pancreatic function.

Recovery depends on the amount of functioning tissue left in the pancreas. When the organs are not destroyed beyond repair, a proper diet and rest will restore normal functioning. It may take a few years.[250]

Airola suggests a lacto-vegetarian, low calorie, alkaline diet of high quality natural foods: plenty of whole grains, especially buckwheat, and raw vegetables and fruits. Contrary to popular belief, fruits are beneficial in the diabetic's diet. Fresh fruits contain fruit sugar, fructose, which does not need insulin for its metabolism and is well tolerated by diabetics.

Complex carbohydrate foods are necessary in the diet of diabetics. The diabetic needs carbohydrates, but they must be natural, unrefined, high-fiber, slow-digesting carbohydrates, such as whole grains, especially buckwheat, millet, and oats. Other examples of complex carbohydrates are corn, rice, squash, pumpkin, potato, pepper, carrots and fruits.

Airola concludes: Emphasis should be on raw foods. About 80 percent of the diet should be raw. Raw foods stimulate the pancreas and increase insulin production.[19, pp70-71]

EARWAX

James Kawchak, MD, writes as follows in the Journal of Occupational Medicine: Earwax, or cerumen, is a very common cause of deafness among Americans. Other symptoms are tinnitus, severe earaches, dizziness, and if the wax gets lodged beyond the isthmus of the ear, it could cause a reflex cough.

Ear wax secreted by our ears lubricates the ear canal, which is prone to infection, and traps bacteria, dust, and insects. It encases foreign objects, then it eliminates them when we are lying down. Usually just talking, yawning, and eating eliminates the wax, but our pabulum diets and the increased pollution in our environment inhibit its natural elimination. Highly processed and boiled foods prevent the jaw motion necessary to remove wax from the ear canal. Chewing raw carrots, celery, apples, and nuts, massage the ear canal in such a way as to move the wax along toward the outer ear. The wax eventually falls out during sleep.

An itchy ear indicates that it is in the process of cleaning out foreign substances along with the wax build-up. But the natural ability of the ear to clean itself can be swamped by environmental smog, dust, or smoke, from which there is no protection.

Many treatments to remove earwax are either useless or downright dangerous. Some prescription drugs, particularly those containing hydrogen peroxide irritate the skin of the ear canal. Neither salt water nor olive oil is effective.[69]

At one time, propylene glycol was thought effective, but in 1947 it was tested by B. H. Senturia and his colleagues. The chemical was found to cause rapid swelling of the wax, which could produce severe pressure and pain and would, of course, make removal of wax more difficult. Water, too, often does more harm than good by causing the wax to swell rapidly.[70]

Kawchak advises that one should refrain from using a cotton swab, because frequent contact with the tympanic membrane can cause the build-up of a delicate callous, which nature then tries to remove. With continued use of a cotton swab to ease itching, a vicious cycle begins that eventually builds on the tympanic membrane a hard callous that results in severe degradation of hearing. The medical field refers to this self-induced damage as "Q-Tip Syndrome." Using swabs for this purpose is unnecessary, since any wax that can be dislocated thereby is on its way to falling out of the ear of its own accord. Harder wax is only compacted more deeply into the ear by pressing the swab against it.

Carmen adds to the "Q-Tip Syndrome" by telling of one of his elderly patients who was watching TV while using a cotton swab. When the phone rang he put the receiver to his ear, forgetting to remove the cotton swab first. The cotton swab punctured the eardrum, breaking the delicate middle ear bones and lodging in the inner ear structure (the cochlea). The fluid of the inner ear escaped, producing instant and permanent deafness in that ear.[12, pp141-142]

HIGH BLOOD PRESSURE, ARTERIOSCLEROSIS, ATHEROSCLEROSIS, HARDENING OF THE ARTERIES, POOR CIRCULATION

Lamb states that high blood pressure may cause tinnitus, affecting both ears. Noise caused by atherosclerosis or high blood pressure is usually high-pitched.

Fatty cholesterol deposits that occur in arteries may obstruct blood circulation to the ear or to the region between the ear and brain. This disturbance of blood flow can induce noise. When the carotid arteries in the neck develop fatty cholesterol, one may hear a "swishing" sound that pulsates with the heartbeat. Usually the source of this sound can be verified by applying pressure against these arteries, which should temporarily eliminate it.[3, p2]

Williams explains the condition of atherosclerosis. As we age, the insides of the blood vessels tend to accumulate deposits which impede blood flow to every part of the body. This makes it harder for the cells and tissues to get the oxygen and nutrients that the blood carries.

These encrustation (plaques) are fatty in nature, but as they become more established they come to contain mineral matter (calcium) and become hard. This is referred to as "hardening of the arteries." Cholesterol was thought to be the cause of these fatty deposits, but cholesterol not only is essential for the functioning of our bodies, it is also produced in our bodies and has functions associated with the very best of health.

If we were to consume less cholesterol, we would sacrifice good nutrition since most of our good foods contain substantial amounts of cholesterol. The evidence shows that good nutrition prevents cholesterol deposits from forming, even when our cholesterol consumption is moderately high.

Williams explains that cholesterol is made within our bodies, and this "homemade" cholesterol can be deposited in the arteries of a person who consumes no cholesterol at all. Furthermore, the rate of production of cholesterol in the body depends upon the supply of cholesterol from the outside. Not consuming cholesterol may in effect "open the valve" which increases production of cholesterol within the body thereby, increasing total cholesterol in the blood stream.[20, pp73-74]

Airola states that high blood pressure is not a disease, but a body's corrective measure initiated to cope with pathological conditions such as general toxemia, impaired kidney function, glandular disturbances, defective calcium metabolism, degenerative changes in arteries (arteriosclerosis), obesity, emotionally-caused dysfunction in the vasomotor mechanism, etc. High blood pressure develops from one or a combination of the following: cigarette smoking, insufficient physical exercise, high levels of cholesterol and blood fats, wrong diet, poor control of diabetes (if present), or inability to deal with emotional stress.

Airola suggests the avoidance of all animal products (except goat's milk), coffee, alcohol, salt, and all strong spices, especially mustard, black and white pepper, ginger, nutmeg, etc.

Eat plenty of raw green leafy vegetables and raw fruits. Watermelons are beneficial. Russian research showed that garlic and buckwheat are good in reducing high blood pressure.[19, p109]

HYPERACUSIS

Hyperacusis is an increased sensitivity to moderate-level environmental sound when hearing thresholds are normal. In the clinical neurologic history, the examiner questions the patient to differentiate sensitivity to sound from that of intolerance to sound. Usually, the tinnitus patient reporting hyperacusis reports "exceptional hearing" before the onset of tinnitus. Hyperacusis is an extremely rare disorder which may affect less than 1 per 100,000 people.[71, p268]

Dan Malcore of The Hyperacusis Network* writes in his newsletter that children with autism have hyperacute hearing. Hyperacute hearing in the autistic child is not the result of a noise injury. That alone makes it very different from hyperacusis. Auditory Training has been helpful in resolving hyperacute hearing in some autistic children. At this point, Auditory Training has not helped the hyperacusis/tinnitus patient, and some patients claim it has actually worsened their condition.

Dan suggests using Desensitization by listening only to frequencies the sufferer is sensitive to. This would involve specific evaluation for personal tapes. Another method would be to desensitize one day at a time, using ear protection when necessary. Pink noise is one way of accomplishing this. Jack Vernon has pink noise tapes. The filter from 6000 band and above. If you wish to buy a tape, call Jack Vernon in Portland, Oregon at 503-494-8032.

It is also possible that the body is deficient in particular vitamins or nutrients.

Dan makes many suggestions in his newsletter on how to keep noise to a minimum. Some of the suggestions include special lavatory faucets that work like a bubbler. Put heavy felt cushions on all the kitchen cabinets and drawers so they are not banging when being closed. Try to deactivate the beep on your microwave. The ideal heat for a home is hot-water-baseboard heat. Find a vacuum cleaner with 1-2 horsepower. (Of course the best vacuum cleaner would be a central vacuum with the motor in a noise-insulated cabinet outside the house.

Ed.) Ranch homes are more desirable than multi-level homes. Central air conditioners are by far the best.

The quietest tire is Goodyear Eagle GA radials. Disconnect the bell ringer on cars for signaling seat belt buckling.

If you have trouble talking on the telephone, get a Handset Amplifier from Radio Shack. The name is a misnomer. This gadget plugs into any phone. It has a volume control and a tone control. If you reduce the volume and tone control all the way down, the normal ear can hardly hear anyone talking on the other end. Radio Shack also offers a Sound Level Meter. You can use the meter for buying various household appliances. There is much information about selecting ear plugs and ear muffs in the newsletter.

Do not have a dentist use an ultrasound cleaner. When it hits the teeth it emits an extremely high-pitched, sharp, loud noise.

Dan claims that drugs are a possible culprit for some of the ear problems, and the only safe general pain reliever is acetaminophen (Tylenol). One reader experienced hyperacusis after receiving metrizamide dye during a routine study of his spine. Dan suggests refraining from caffeinated beverages, alcohol, and chocolate. Hyperacusis has also been noted in some females during certain stages of the menstrual cycle, in some patients with anxiety disorders, Williams syndrome, early Menière's disease, Bell's palsy, or certain endocrine and metabolic disorders.[72]

There is a homeopathic remedy that might be helpful in reducing the sensitivity to sound. The company sells it to health professionals only, except in certain areas of the country where there are no therapists to prescribe it. The product is called Formula N. It is available from:

Terrace International Distributors, Inc.
P.O. Box 817
Forest Falls, CA 92339
(909) 794-7674
(800) 824-2434

IMPACTED WISDOM TOOTH

Roy E. Bean, M.D., stated that many hearing problems are a result of a nerve blocking due to tooth impaction or crowded teeth. Anything that causes a nerve blocking can cause ringing ears. It may take several weeks after removal of the tooth for any relief of the tinnitus. Bean suggests using "pointed pressure therapy."[73, p187]

INFECTIONS AND INFLAMMATIONS

Labyrinthitis, an inflammation of the inner ear, occurs when the inner ear is invaded by any one of a variety of germs from diseases present elsewhere in the body, such as meningitis, syphilis, and various other types of infections.

When pus is present, the sensory elements of the cochlea can be destroyed, resulting in permanent loss of hearing.

Viral labyrinthitis is most often due to mumps, influenza, and measles, and mumps is regarded as the most common cause of unilateral (one sided) deafness in children. Medical care should be obtained immediately.[4, pp100-101]

Andrew Freeland warns in his book, Deafness: The Facts, that the removal of wax eliminates the barrier to infection and creates trauma. Even when done with soft cotton buds. And trying to flush the wax from the ears by using modified syringes will only dissolve the ear's greasy, protective lining which ultimately will lead to infection. Soapy water in the ear-canal changes the pH (acidity level) to an alkaline state, which again removes the natural bacterial and fungal barrier to infection.[74]

LOW BLOOD PRESSURE/HYPOGLYCEMIA

Low blood pressure can produce tinnitus, but it is usually mild, and varies in frequency.[3, p2]

Rodale points out that the medical community views low blood pressure as a blessing, for if you have it you will probably never be afflicted with all the unpleasant symptoms of high blood pressure. But there are a few exceptions: Addison's disease, poor nutrition, low basal metabolism, or hypothyroidism (a thyroid gland which does not send out enough of the gland secretion). Postural hypotension is an extreme case of low blood pressure where the individual faints or blacks out from a sudden change in posture.

Rodale claims that many of these conditions are due to poor nutrition.[6, pp223-225]

The ear has one of the most delicate circulation

networks and one of the highest energy requirements in comparison to other systems in the body. Hypoglycemia decreases the amount of energy-releasing glucose that reaches the ear and is frequently the sole cause of tinnitus.[75]

Excess refined sugars can lead to hypoglycemia. Sugar also weakens the adrenal glands and disrupts the sodium/potassium balance throughout the body, including the delicate organs of the middle ear. This alone often results in tinnitus and hearing difficulties.[76]

In addition to eliminating refined sugars and saturated fats (which block small blood vessels), certain nutrients have been shown to help tinnitus by increasing the blood flow and oxygen in the inner ear. Suggested nutrients are omega-3 fatty acids (eat fatty fish, such as mackerel and salmon, three or four times a week, or take fish oil capsules -- 3 mg daily). Improvement should result within six weeks. The B-vitamin niacin helps by causing the small blood vessels to dilate or open up (take 100 to 1500 mg daily).[77]

MÉNIÈRE'S DISEASE

This affliction involves hemorrhaging of the small, delicate parts of the inner ear. According to Family Medical Guide the disease may be the result of any or all of the following: acute or chronic infection, otosclerosis, trauma associated with brain concussion, hardening of the arteries, congenital malformations of the inner ear, allergy, toxins, and blood disorders such as leukemia. Any or all of these possible causes of the inner ear disorder may result from aging. Some in the medical profession suggest as two causes an imbalance of fluid and pressure in the inner ear or an electrolyte (mineral) imbalance. The disease is characterized by sudden intermittent attacks of spinning vertigo, dizziness, tinnitus, nausea, vomiting, and partial deafness. The attacks are sporadic.[78]

The Encyclopedia Britannica adds a few more causes: intense heat and exposure to the sun, rheumatism, influenza, venereal disease, anemia and leukemia. The attacks of vertigo tend to become less frequent, and may entirely elapse, but the deafness may remain permanent.[79]

The latest surgical treatment for Ménière's disease, called RVN, was developed by Herbert Silverstein, MD, president of the Ear Research Foundation in Sarasota, Florida, according to a 1987 article in Parade magazine. Before surgery, a small, custom made earphone that produces a predetermined pattern of steady auditory clicks is clipped to the outer ear. An incision is made behind the ear to expose the vestibular and cochlear nerves, and an electrode from a nearby video monitor is placed on the cochlear nerve to sense the signals being transmitted through the cochlear nerve after having passed through the inner ear. The pattern of nerve impulses is compared on the monitor with the pattern piped into the source earphone. A difference in the two patterns indicates a possible injury to the hearing nerve. The fibers of the vestibular nerve are then severed layer by layer until the response pattern on the cochlear matches that of the input stimulus.[80]

Hundreds of surgeons have been trained to perform this operation. For more information write:

Ear Research Foundation*

James T. Spencer, MD, of West Virginia put one of his patients on a wholesome diet in an attempt to alleviate his Ménière's disease, eliminating all of the following: salt, refined sugar, foods with added sugar, processed foods and beverages, desserts, cream, and fatty meats. Foods with concentrated sweetness—prunes, figs, dates, and honey—were reduced. The diet consisted only of fresh foods: lean meat, poultry, fish, dairy products, fruits, vegetables, and whole grain breads and cereals. He reports that after three weeks, the patient had only one dizzy spell and began to regain his hearing. After six weeks his hearing greatly improved.[81]

Fry expands on Spencer's view of Ménière's disease in his response to a woman in his advisory newsletter. The writer complains of hot sweats, dizziness, headaches, whirling vertigo, vomiting and excessive bowel movements.

Fry answered that Ménière's disease progressively evolves into tinnitus and deafness. He warns against using any medications because they can complicate and worsen the problem.

Fry asserted that the woman's problem was caused by saturation of the body and labyrinths of the ear with toxic materials. This causes irritation and may cause the body's "gyrocompass" to fail or function, thus causing staggering and falling.

The causes of toxicity are, among others, consumption of cooked foods, foods contrary to man's biological disposition, incorrectly combined foods, condiments and seasonings, etc.

Fry suggested that she consider fasting for two to

four weeks, conditioning the body to detoxify itself and repair damages it may have sustained.[25p]

Three drugs that have been advocated by many for Ménière's syndrome are histamine, potassium iodide, and ammonium chloride.[82]

OTOSCLEROSIS

Otosclerosis is a formation of a bone overgrowth in the region of the oval window, immobilizing the stapes bone. The stapes transmits sound vibrations from the tympanic membrane across the ear to the inner ear fluids. The impairment of its piston-like movement produces a gradual conductive hearing loss.

This hearing loss usually begins in the 20s and 30s, is more common in women than men, and often develops during pregnancy. In about half of the cases, there is a positive family history. The hearing loss is gradual and progressive, ultimately affecting both ears. It rarely progresses to complete deafness. Victims can usually hear well over the telephone with amplification. A hearing aid can help, but surgery is preferable because it is usually successful.

An operation called a stapedectomy is performed under local anesthesia through the ear canal. After the tympanic membrane is elevated, the stapes bone is removed and a prosthesis—a piston or a tiny bit of wire—is inserted into the oval window. Hearing returns immediately. The chances of success are better than 90 percent.[24, pp290-291]

Another source states that the disease is often

accompanied by tinnitus, and sometimes by vertigo. There is also a difference of opinion as to the success of stapedectomy, with some claiming that the operation is usually performed on only one ear at a time because there is a risk that total deafness may result in the operated ear.[65, p759]

STRESS

The auditory (hearing) pathway is one of the most delicate and sensitive mechanisms of the human body. Since it is directly linked with the general nervous system, its responses are in direct proportion to the person's state of anxiety. (Ed.)

Patricia R. House, MD, declares that tinnitus can be a stress-related disorder. As the person is faced with dissension, physiological changes occur as a result of the "fight or flight" reaction. Personality and the ability to cope are related to the patient's perceptions of the tinnitus. The constant pressure from varying states of stress and distress in modern life can cause the patient to be constantly mobilized for action (a rigidifying of neuromuscular systems). This mobilization can be responsible for the onset or exacerbation of a tinnitus episode.

Tinnitus is a stressful experience, and even more stress is generated by the cause of the noise. A patient's disturbance from tinnitus may vary from mild irritation to thoughts of suicide. This range represents differences arising from the patient's coping mechanisms, personality defense structure, social factors, the severity of the tinnitus, and related otological problems.

Attitude helps to determine the threshold for pain and disturbance. Attention is drawn towards the body and bodily functions. When tests reveal that there is no serious medical problem, many patients stop worrying and the stress is relieved.[83]

John J. Shea, MD, observed that patients with chronic intractable pain are psychologically similar to the patient with chronic intractable tinnitus—rigid, obsessive, neurotic, insecure, chronically fatigued and depressed.[84]

My physician remarked to me that stress can restrict the flow of blood to the inner ear.

For people whose tinnitus increases with, or is linked to stress, spiritual, self-help books and tapes are available that may have a calming effect. The book, You Can Heal Your Life, by Louise L. Hay, was found most helpful by those with the described characteristics in the self-help group.[85]

Another excellent book is The Relaxation Response, by Herbert Benson.[86]

TMJ SYNDROME

Marshall Lubin, DC, explains that TMJ stands for temporomandibular joint. He states that TMJ syndrome is frequently associated with automobile accidents. Symptoms that may arise following these accidents include: headaches, neck pain, back pain, pain during chewing, insomnia, tinnitus and jaw pain. Pain upon opening of the mouth is known as the Number One indicator of TMJ Dysfunction.

The temporomandibular joint is a sliding-hinge joint. It is located where the temple and the lower jaw joint meet.

Treatment of TMJ syndrome may vary. Inflammation is usually present, requiring an anti-inflammatory medication. Pulsed ultrasound over the joint also helps to reduce inflammation and clear any fluid that may have accumulated in the joint.

Ultrasound and manual massage of the affected muscles help to reduce spasm. Chiropractic manipulation of the upper back and neck reduces dislocations in the spinal segments that become dislocated due to stress.[87]

Dixie Farley, writing for FDA/Consumer, adds: also commonly reported are various joint noises, which may or may not be sign of a TM disorder. A click when opening the jaw may indicate a displaced disk, but many people have noises without having a TM disorder. A grating or crackling noise more likely signifies arthritis. Moreover, not all TM patients have joint noises. Joint noises without pain or restricted jaw movement would not be enough evidence for a diagnosis of a TM disorder.

More than 26 TMJ therapies are in use, by one estimate, and treatment is given not only by dentists, physicians, and oral surgeons but also by persons outside traditional dentistry and medicine, such as psychologists and chiropractors.

Whenever possible, TMJ-disorder therapies should be conservative and reversible. Such measures bring symptomatic relief to 80 percent of patients. Therapy usually lasts about three months.

This article also presents the benefits and drawbacks of four radiological tests for TMJ disorders. Those four are: 1) Ordinary X-rays, 2) Arthrography, 3) Computed Tomography (CT), 4) Magnetic Resonance Imaging (MRI).[88]

A dentist or orthodontist can eliminate the symptoms of TMJ with the aid of a myomonitor, an electronic device that helps locate the position of the lower jaw in relation to the upper jaw. Once this occlusal (bite) analysis is performed, an appliance is installed on the lower teeth to relieve the spasm and thereby eliminate the symptoms. By means of the myomonitor in conjunction with a kinesiograph (an oscilloscope tracking device), the exact position of the mandible (lower jaw) can be recorded for all future reconstruction work.[89]

Prevention magazine excerpted the following from Andrew Kaplan's book Self-Help for TMJ: suggests the following self-help modalities: One way to control the pain of inflammation is to avoid coffee. Caffeine stimulates the central nervous system, increases muscle tension, and increases sensitivity to pain.

Limit jaw movement. Open your jaws only as far as you experience no pain. If you feel a yawn coming, prevent it by pressing a fist under your chin.

Eat a soft diet. For main dishes, use pasta, fish, eggs, and minced meat. Eat cooked vegetables instead of raw. Avoid nuts, hard rolls, and chewy meat. Don't chew gum.

Apply heat to the jaw area by using hot cloths, a heating pad, or a hot water bottle.

Also available are professional devices such as the Hydrocolator, available at hospital-supply stores and some drug stores. It contains a fluid-filled plastic pouch that is inserted into a fabric wrapper held in place with Velcro fasteners.

Some people respond better to the application of cold to the jaw area. Don't apply ice for more than about 20 minutes in any hour or you can damage your skin. (My dentist uses a soft rubber glove filled with frozen corn or peas. It is soft and flexible).

Correct bad posture. Don't position your head with the head thrust forward and the chin tilted up. Don't stand in an exaggerated military posture. Don't sit in a slumped position or cross-legged or for a long time in one position without a break. When driving, keep the seat comfortably close to the dashboard. Don't sleep on your stomach. Don't cradle the telephone between your shoulder and chin. Don't carry a heavy shoulder bag on the same shoulder for an extended period. Don't wear high-heeled boots or shoes.

Break the teeth-clenching habit. Retrain your body's whole response to stress by using stress therapy, psychotherapy and biofeedback.[90]

Another excellent book is TMJ: The Self-Help Program. You might find it in the public library.[91] For more information about TMJ, see ADDENDUM of this book.

VIRUSES

Almost any of the common infectious diseases of childhood, which in general are viral rather than bacterial, may in severe cases, affect the inner ear, according to the book Hearing and Deafness.[92]

As we learned earlier, loss of hearing precedes tinnitus.

The following diseases are human viral diseases:

1. Major epidemic diseases: small pox, yellow fever and typhous.
2. Common specific infectious diseases: measles, mumps, chicken pox (with its variant form of herpes zoster, shingles), rubella or "German measles."
3. Rarer infections, mostly derived from animals: rabies and several forms of encephalitis.[79, 23:191a]

Other viruses are: meningitis, mononucleosis, diphtheria, scarlet fever, influenza, viral hepatitis, and, polio.[1-p2564, 4-p127, 92-pp121-122, 93]

The book Hearing and Deafness continues: frequently, as is usual with mumps, only one ear is damaged, but all too often both ears suffer. A virus may severely injure delicate specialized structures such as the organ of Corti and the tectorial membrane in the inner ear.

There is no hope of regeneration or repair of a missing organ of Corti. And no type of treatment, medication, or stimulation will improve the hearing of anyone whose deafness is due to toxic degeneration to viral infections such as mumps and measles, which also cause severe and permanent structural changes.

Freese explains that if children suffer severe viral infections (such as viral meningitis) during the first year of life, their hearing may be partially or entirely destroyed, just as viral infections destroy hearing during the prenatal period.[4, p127]

Freese continues: about 10 percent of congenital deafness is the result of prenatal rubella infections. The development of rubella vaccine has considerably reduced the incidence of the disease and the number of hearing-impaired children. Hopefully, further research will provide vaccines or other measures to control the damage of the aforementioned viral diseases. Certainly prospective mothers should keep informed of such new developments in preventive medicine and take advantage of them.

Although viral infections cannot be satisfactorily treated yet, many of the serious ones can be prevented. Smallpox, for example, has been totally eradicated through a combination of vaccination and isolation of cases. It is also possible to vaccinate against measles, German measles, yellow fever, polio and rabies.[1, p2567]

The same source states that the basic structure of viruses is so simple that it is questionable whether they should be regarded as living matter at all. Essentially they consist of no more than a capsule of protein which contains their genetic material in the form of one of the nucleic acids, DNA or RNA—the substances which carry the genetic message from generation to generation in all living things.[1, p2565]

Perhaps that is why there is disagreement by some in the medical field regarding the safety of vaccinations. Again, my purpose of writing this book is to present you with all the material found even if they are controversial. I do not stand in judgment of them.

E. McBean, Phd, PhD, ND, has written a book titled, Vaccinations Do Not Protect. Some of his arguments are: the medical field refuses to guarantee vaccines; vaccines cause disease—they do not protect; no immunity is developed from vaccination; germs, viruses, etc. do not cause disease. McBean cites world reports on vaccine disasters.[25q]

Biological phenomena tend to occur along a continuum, and if vaccinations can cause death and other disabilities, they also might cause many milder disorders in greater numbers of people. So theorizes Harris L. Coulter, Ph.D., author of the book Vaccination, Social Violence and Criminology: The Medical Assault on the American Brain.

Since the compulsory vaccination of children, cancer has now increased to such frightening proportions that it's the number one killer of children under 15 years of age. Heart disease is the number one killer of adults; TB is on the rise; mental disease is at an all-time high.

In his book, Dr. Coulter suggests that vaccinations have produced widespread brain damage resulting in a host of developmental disabilities and sociopathic problems affecting large numbers of American children. He estimates that one in five children or six is damaged to some degree by vaccinations.

Dr. Coulter's research led him to believe the

following physical symptoms of vaccination damage can include: sub-average IQ loss, vision problems including dyslexia, partial loss of hearing, chronic earaches, asthma or other breathing difficulties, sleep disturbances, allergies, hyperactivity, and lowered resistance to infection. There can also be mental and emotional problems, such as paranoia, low self-esteem, anxiety, autism, depression, sexual precociousness, substance abuse, fascination with fire, outbursts of rage, and lack of remorse.[94]

There is definitely some validity in McBean's book. An AP Wire Service, date lined Washington, DC, told of a toll-free hot line being set up to tell people about federal compensation for those injured by vaccinations. The hot line was part of the Health Resources and Services Administration' s efforts to publicize an October 1st, 1990, deadline for claims against the National Vaccine Injury Compensation Program.

The program provided compensation for injuries from vaccines for diphtheria, tetanus, pertussis (whooping cough), measles, mumps, rubella and polio.[editor]

The federal government has mandated that brochures about the risks and benefits associated with infant vaccination be distributed to parents in every clinic and pediatric office throughout the country. Parents must read the brochures before their children are vaccinated. (Ed.)

STREPTOCOCCUS PNEUMONIA

Hulda Regehr Clark states in her book Cure For All Diseases that tinnitus is caused by three things acting in partnership: toxic elements, an allergy to *salicylates* (the aspirin family) and a bacterium *Streptococcus pneumoniae* (the pneumonia bug). This "bug" can be carried in the chronic state after a bout of pneumonia or what seems to be a head cold. It is always present in an earache. The strep bug can also cause *Meniere's syndrome*.

Streptococcus pneumoniae often hides in pockets under infected teeth and in holes left where teeth have been pulled-- especially wisdom teeth. These can be found by alternative dentists who clean these cavitations. *Strep* also resides in the liver; clean them out with liver flushes. (This is explained in her book. See BOOKS in RESOURCE section).

Clark also recommends avoiding exposure to certain toxic elements--lead, beryllium, zirconium, benzalkonium. They are present in the environment at gas stations and in many of our body lotions, soaps and salves. (This is all explained in her book. I highly recommend it.)

PHYSIOLOGICAL INTERVENTION

The reason why some of the following therapies are effective, is that tinnitus might have some of its origins in a dysfunction of some mechanical component of the body, as the muscular-skeletal system. This sections describes those therapies.

ACUPRESSURE

Acupressure is based on promoting health by stimulating energy, using pressure on the skin at various points along meridians associated with the function of vital organs.

Acupressure is like acupuncture without needles. It is essentially a self-help technique in which the fingers are used to apply pressure to points known to be helpful for relief of various types of pain. It is particularly good for stress disorders and for improving energy.[96]

One woman in the group could hear a pulsating sound or a continuous hum in her left ear. She was told by her acupressurist to apply gentle compression on the jugular vein, which alleviated the sound.

Another source states that acupressure was discovered by the Chinese more than five thousand years ago. They found that therapeutic benefits are obtained through the "unblocking" of various pathways to specific body points of the body.

Massage the points shown below which relate to tinnitus problems for at least 5 minutes the first day increasing to 8 minutes twice a day. Use your thumb and apply vigorous (but not painful) pressure to those areas.

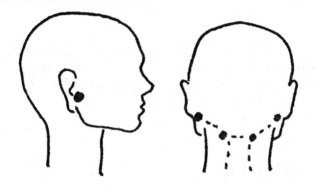

ACUPUNCTURE

Acupuncture can be described as a branch of Chinese medicine in which needles are used to puncture the skin at certain defined points in order to restore the balance of energy, as therapy for various disorders, or to induce anesthesia. [65-p66, 95-pp120-121]

Traditional Chinese medicine holds that the Chi (life force) flows through the body along meridians (channels); blockage in one or more of these meridians is believed to cause ill health. Acupuncturists aim to restore health by inserting needles at appropriate sites, known as acupuncture points, on the affected meridians.

Research suggests that acupuncture causes the release within the central nervous system of morphine like substances, endorphins, which act as natural analgesics (pain killers).[65, p66]

The following experiment was performed by N. J. Marks, at Guy's Hospital in London; First he noted that there are similarities in the mechanisms of pain and tinnitus. Within the auditory system, well-established pathways exist that could constitute a reflex arc. Two-way pathways connect the brainstem nuclei to the reticular formation, the thalamus, and the cortex. This arrangement has marked similarities to the unusual neural pathways found in the mediation of pain. There, one finds elaborate feedback loops that, when activated, are capable of reducing the intensity of persistent pain.

In light of these similarities, he wondered what acupuncture might have to offer the tinnitus sufferer. The mechanism of acupuncture currently hypothesized is that it stimulates the body's endogenous (generated within the body) opiates, which work both centrally and at a local level. The question struck him: Will these opiates suppress tinnitus as well as pain?

He selected 14 patients with chronic tinnitus and for four weeks administered a weekly 20-minute treatment of electro-acupuncture with alternating low and high frequencies. On the group as a whole he found little general effect, but five patients reported noticing a subjective improvement. Marks was reluctant to close the door on this harmless treatment and disparage it outright, suggesting that there are some sufferers who may respond to courses longer than two weeks.[96]

BREATHING EXERCISES

One of the most effective techniques I found to reduce the intensity of my tinnitus is alternate nostril breathing, which I learned from taking a yoga class. After a minute or two of this exercise, you will be able to hear little "air pops" in the middle ear, a manifestation of the freer exchange of air. The exercise will result in a vigorous dislodging and subsequent removal of accumulated pollutants in the ear canal. It is done in two steps. The third and fourth steps are contingency steps in case of blockage.

1. Breathe naturally in through both nostrils. Breath out through one nostril, pressing the other one closed.
2. Press one nostril closed and breathe in and out through the other.
3. If one nostril is blocked, press it closed and breathe in through the one that is less closed. Then press the freer nostril closed and try to breathe out through the other one.
4. If both nostrils are blocked, breathe in through your mouth and try to breathe out through the less blocked nostril. If that nostril opens sufficiently to allow it, breathe in and out through it and stop mouth breathing.

Perform this exercise twice a day for five minutes or as often as you like. After you have found relief from the tinnitus, once a day may be sufficient for maintenance.

CHIROPRACTIC

Chiropractic is a health care science that deals with the vital relationship between the nervous system and the spinal column and with the role of this relationship in the rehabilitation and maintenance of health. An unobstructed flow of nerve impulses from the brain through the spinal nerves and onward to every body cell helps achieve the balance, harmony, and vitality we need to enjoy vibrant health

110

and a long, productive life.[97]

Obviously trauma to the ear, either from loud noises, or a direct blow can leave permanent damage as well as start tinnitus problems. Even injury to the neck can be a cause. The lower portion of the brain stem actually descends into the area of the first two vertebra or bones in the spine. Misalignments of these vertebrae (called subluxations) can cause nerve interference and result in tinnitus. Specific chiropractic adjustments in this area have stopped thousands of long-standing tinnitus problems.[98]

If you do seek out a chiropractor, try to find one who follows the principles of natural hygiene. I have listed them under NATURAL HYGIENIST, current as of August 1991. For an updated list of natural hygienists who are also chiropractors in your area, send a business-size self-addressed stamped envelope to Victoria Bidwell.[99]

CLEARING A BLOCKED EUSTACHIAN TUBE

A blocked eustachian tube may bring on a flare of tinnitus because air on the throat side of the eardrum becomes trapped and can no longer vary in pressure to keep up with the changes in atmospheric pressure external to the eardrum. Relief may be obtained by means of what is known as the Valsalva maneuver. This is the forcible exhalation (or inhalation) effort against a closed glottis (the cleft between the vocal cords and the larynx). To do this, close your mouth, pinch your nostrils shut and try to exhale (or inhale) gently until the eardrum pressure equalizes and restores your hearing to normal. Be careful. Don't attempt this if you have a cold or flu, because you can blow germs into the sinuses and middle ears. If your nose gets stuffy from this maneuver, perform the yoga breathing exercises described above.[editor]

111

EAR MASSAGE

Carmen states that in some cases of sensorineural hearing loss, (remember, tinnitus is a precursor of hearing loss) patients have insisted that they hear better if they press on the skull behind the ear, or tilt the head, or apply pressure to the neck.

Ear massage cannot restore hearing in a clinically diagnosed case of nerve deafness. In this case, the eustachian tube does not function to equalize pressure in the middle ear cavity, and therefore rubbing the ear gently, yawning, swallowing, chewing, rotating the jaw, or holding the nose closed while trying to blow through it can fill the middle ear with the needed air. This can not be accomplished in an altitudinal change. Carmen cautions that ear massage can result in a separation of the joints of the middle ear bones (malleus, incus or stapes) and can be dangerous.[12, p79]

ELECTRICAL/MAGNETIC STIMULATION

Transcutaneous and transpromontory electrical stimulation has been described for the treatment of tinnitus. The Department of Otolaryngology, Otsu Red Cross Hospital, Shiga, Japan, has been using cochlear implantation to relieve tinnitus. Doctors implanted cochlear implants in twenty patients since 1987. Electrical stimulation was used which resulted in relief of tinnitus in 72% of the patients.[100]

Ellis Douek, MD, of London, also is experimenting with electrical suppression of tinnitus. In a modification of the cochlear implant that may make it feasible for tinnitus patients, he implants an electrode against the round window of the inner ear. This procedure may be the ultimate key to electrical suppression of tinnitus, since it provides a current path through the inner ear.

The report also tells about A. Morgan, MD, in Lyon, France, who has developed an instrument called the Tintip. It delivers 144-Hz synchronous electrical and sound pulses to the ear. Each stimulus is set at a maximum comfort level. The treatment lasts for 45 minutes and is repeated every ten days, for a total of six treatments. Morgan reports a 54 percent success rate with this procedure.[7e]

Colin Kemp, an Australian engineer, markets a unit he calls the Tinnitus Inhibitor, a pocket-sized battery-operated device that generates a variety of pure tones. Patients adjust the tone control until they find the tone that most nearly matches the primary pitch of their tinnitus. For a short time they then use an earpiece to introduce that tone to the tinnitus ear at an intensity that masks the tinnitus. The tinnitus usually is reduced for a brief period after the masking tone is turned off.[7f]

For more information on the work of Douek, Morgan, or Kemp, write to the American Tinnitus Association.*

HEARING AIDS

Lamb wrote in one of his syndicated columns that any measure that improves hearing often suppresses tinnitus. A person may not be aware of a hearing loss because it involves sound frequencies that are not in the range of normal conversation. These usually involve loss of high frequency hearing. The ear noise may be in those same frequencies. In such cases, the hearing aid is not so much to improve hearing as to stop the tinnitus.

Freese notes that about 225,000 of the hearing aids purchased yearly are bought directly from a commercial hearing-aid vendor. Vendors are neither equipped nor trained to do a proper hearing-aid evaluation, to adequately train the patient in the use of the device, or to carry out the aural rehabilitation necessary. This results in nearly half of the aids so purchased being unnecessary and inappropriate.

Before you consider purchasing a hearing aid, you should be examined by both an otologist and an audiologist. If the two agree, then the audiologist will do a hearing-aid evaluation to find out whether a hearing aid will be of help to you.[4, pp144-145]

Three people out of nine in our tinnitus group claimed that a hearing aid provided the greatest relief from tinnitus.

Various government agencies can help you if you have an unresolved dispute with the dispenser. I have listed them in RESOURCES under Hearing Aids.

HEAT/COLD

Hot and cold therapy can palliate your tinnitus. Use a moist heating pad. If you don't have one, a hot, wet towel under your regular heating pad is effective. After a few minutes, change to a cold compress, again for just a few minutes. Drug stores now sell a soft, flexible vinyl bag that is ideal for these treatments. You can either freeze the bag for cold compresses or place it in boiling water for hot compresses.[editor]

I have already mentioned using a soft surgical glove filled with frozen corn or peas. This will form around the ear comfortably.

HYPNOTHERAPY

McFadden reports that there is no known large-scale

114

study on the effectiveness of hypnosis on tinnitus. Two cases were reported in 1973 in which relief was obtained following hypnosis. In both instances, the primary problem was interference with sleep.

One patient was instructed in a "mind over matter" approach while under hypnosis to concentrate on the tinnitus and note that its intensity was diminishing. Posthypnotic suggestion was given so that the patient could do this himself at bedtime with the same effect. Over a 6-week span the patient found that the tinnitus was greatly subdued.

The second patient was told, under hypnosis, to recall a favorite musical passage whenever his tinnitus became annoying. The stated intent of this was to create an internally generated masking sound for the tinnitus, which proved effective.

McFadden concluded that hypnosis is a viable therapy, and that the patient could produce a feeling of control over the symptom, thus supplying a sense of relief.[36, pp83-84]

MASKING

Tinnitus maskers (Figure 4) have been used to drown out tinnitus. These units, which look like hearing aids, generate a band of white noise piped into the patient's ear. The principle here is that the masking sound is a substitute for the tinnitus sound. The masking sound is an external sound and as such can be much more easily ignored than the internal sound of tinnitus.[7g]

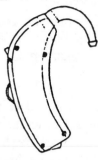

A TINNITUS MASKER

A masker probably will look like a hearing aid. Sometimes a masker and hearing aid occupy the same case and this is called a tinnitus instrument.

Figure 4: Source: American Tinnitus Association. Portland, Oregon.

Robert W. Baloh in his book <u>Dizziness, Hearing Loss, and Tinnitus</u> recommends that the band width of the masking noise be tailored to the patient's tinnitus. Hearing amplification and masking can be combined in the same unit, so that patients with significant hearing loss and tinnitus may also be helped by masking.

As a general rule, the louder the masker must be set the less effective it will be. Thus, the first step in fitting a masking unit is to identify a sound that effectively masks the tinnitus at the lowest sensation level.

One dramatic result of tinnitus masking is the production of residual inhibition, that is, variable duration of suppression of tinnitus after the masking sound is removed. Residual inhibition occurs in most patients, but unfortunately it usually lasts only a brief time.

Baloh continues: The most extensive program involving maskers for tinnitus sufferers involved 493 patients over a 3-year period. Of the 380 patients for whom an instrument was recommended, 158 were still wearing the instrument after a period of time ranging from 1 to 3 years.

Many of the patients reported that their tinnitus was

116

masked, but they rejected the device because the noise was objectionable. Newer tinnitus maskers with high-frequency transducers, narrow bands of noise, and low output may improve patient acceptance of these units. [101, pp172-173]

Lamb suggests you use your radio as a masker if your tinnitus keeps you awake. Place the radio near the bed. Tune it between stations on FM, so that you get a hissing noise. Then turn up the volume. Lamb claims this will work for about two-thirds of the sufferers. [3, p4]

The Craigwell Company, in Dorchester, England, produces a tinnitus suppressor called the Craigwell Master. It is a rented unit in which the patient custom designs an audio tape with the noise that best masks the sounds heard in his own particular case of tinnitus. [7h]

Also available is a new masking device that has the natural sounds of rain, surf, and waterfalls. You can adjust the frequency and intensity to best drown out your own tinnitus. It weighs less than three pounds, so is convenient for travel. You can connect it to your sound system or plug your headphones into it. For more information, write Ambient Shapes, Inc.* The product's name is Marsona 1200, #TMA 120.

The following information was added in my fourth edition:

Dr. Paul Yanick disagrees with the use of maskers. He states that sound maskers overstimulate the ear to encourage desensitization, and thereby overstress, or further damage already damaged ears.

OSTEOPATHY

An osteopath is a practitioner of medicine and surgery who holds the degree of Doctor of Osteopathy. In addition to using all the procedures of contemporary medical practice, the osteopath stresses the importance of the musculoskeletal system (the bones, muscles, and their connecting tendons and ligaments) in the improvement and maintenance of health. Consequently, special emphasis is placed on body mechanics and manipulative methods of dealing with and treating many illnesses. Osteopathy differs from orthodox medical practice in that it holds to the theory that diseases are caused to a significant degree by the obstruction of nerves and arteries by pressure from all adjusted bones, especially those in the spine. [9, 17:2238-2240]

Leon Chaitow, ND, DO, author of Alternative Therapies: Osteopathy: A Complete Health-Care System, adds the following definition: Within a man's body there exists a constant tendency towards health, if this capacity is recognized and normalized. The structure of the body is reciprocally related to its function. So given the opportunity to mobilize its forces, the body will cure itself. [103]

The following is my experience with osteopathy: One day after working in my vegetable garden, I developed a pain in my back and tried to sooth it by lying awhile in a tub of hot water. I bent my head back to wet my hair, and in desperation to rid myself of the ringing in my ear, I began to massage various areas of my head while partially submerged under the water. After about two minutes I raised my head to find the ringing almost gone! I figured I had touched a particular bone that perhaps took pressure off a nerve and hoped that I had eliminated the ringing for good. It returned the next day.

I tried the position four times after that without favorable results. My osteopath used several methods to relieve my

118

tinnitus, but I only got minor, temporary relief. But even temporary relief is a treatment in the right direction. Another person in the group had the intensity of his noise decrease. So it is certainly worth a try.

I will forewarn you that finding an osteopath is not easy, even though there are over 28,000 osteopathic physicians throughout the 50 states. I have been told that most phone books don't have a specific listing under osteopaths. I have listed the Osteopathic Colleges in the United States under RESOURCES. They can direct you to an osteopath in your area.

See ADDENDUM for further information about Osteopathy.

REFLEXOLOGY

Reflexology is a form of therapeutic foot massage which facilitates healing by improving circulation and nerve function.

The feet are a perfect microcosm of the body. All of the nerves at the sole of the feet are connected to all of the organs in the body. When pressure is applied to certain points on the feet, electro-chemical nerve impulses are activated, forming a "message" to a specific organ.

Reflexology is considered to be a holistic healing technique which aims to treat the individual as a whole in order to induce a state of balance and harmony in body, mind, and spirit. The reflexologist doesn't cure -- only the body has the capacity to cure. What reflexology does is work with the subtle energy flows which revitalize the body so that its own natural healing ability can initiate healing.

Professional massage of the reflex areas on the feet serves

to establish which parts of the body are out of balance and therefore not working efficiently.[102]

One person in the group became involved in reflexology to help her husband improve his hearing. He had lost 60% of his hearing in his right ear due to taking cortisone shots for pain. Several weeks passed before he notice his hearing was impaired. After the first treatment, he checked to see if his hearing improved by putting on his headphones to his electric piano, and found that he was able to hear notes on both sides of the range which he was unable to hear before.

When this first happened, the wife reasoned that since tinnitus is a precursor of hearing loss, perhaps it could help reduce her tinnitus. After only three treatments her tinnitus was reduced to a mellow tone. Eighty percent of her diet was raw food, but when she ate steamed vegetables, she was unable to stop using butter. She knew that the butter was causing a build-up of mucus in her body, which was detrimental to her tinnitus. Finally, her tinnitus was relieved by eliminating the butter and having weekly reflexology treatments.

Reflexology techniques can also be accomplished by anyone. Family members can also help each other. The massage technique for tinnitus is simple, natural and safe.

- Sit in a comfortable chair, sofa, on the bed or floor.
- Cross one of your legs over the other, resting the foot on the opposite knee as shown in picture.
- Massage the foot reflex areas shown below that relate to the ears and the tinnitus condition. Massage for 5 minutes the first day and increase to at least 8 minutes twice a day.

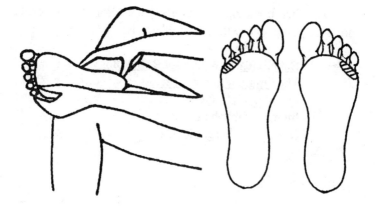

The picture below shows the reflex areas for the ears and tinnitus. When performing the hand reflexology exercises note that your right hand relates to your right ear--and likewise with the left side. Follow the same instructions.

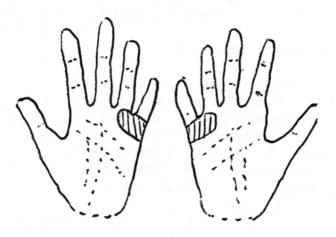

See "Reflexology" in the RESOURCE section for a reflexologist near you.

Another book on the subject that explains the exact pressure points to use for ear problems is:

Better Health With Foot Reflexology:
The Original Ingham Method
by Dwight C. Byers
Ingham Publishing, Inc.
Saint Petersburg, Florida

SURGERY

John House, MD, and Derald Brackmann, MD, explain that surgical treatment of tinnitus includes destructive procedures (removal of the inner-ear structure), neurectomies (cutting a nerve), stapedectomies (removal of stapes), and tympanosympathectomies (sectioning and removal of the tympanic plexus).

In the same source, Dandy (1941) described his experience with tinnitus in 401 patients in whom he sectioned the auditory nerve for Mèniére's disease. He claimed that 50 percent of the patients had an improvement in their tinnitus.

When the hearing of patients is non-serviceable and they are having intractable vertigo, constant dizziness or unsteadiness, the inner-ear structure is removed. Some of the patients who underwent a destructive procedure continued to experience constant unsteadiness or disequilibrium. Postmortem examination of some of these temporal bones revealed traumatic neuromas filling the vestibule.

For some reason, objective tinnitus tends to respond to surgical management better than subjective tinnitus. In cases where objective tinnitus has a venous "hum," relief was accomplished by ligating the internal jugular vein.[76, pp204-208]

Fishbein's Illustrated Medical and Health Encyclopedia describes surgical operations that range from cutting of the nerves to total removal of the labyrinth (inner ear), with which comes total hearing loss. In half of these cases, however, even such surgical procedures did not eliminate the tinnitus.[9, 2602-2603]

Another source states that otosclerosis causes new bone to be laid down around the stirrup bone (stapes), preventing it from transmitting sound properly from the eardrum to the inner ear. When an operation is performed in which the stapes are removed and a plastic replacement fitted, hearing is restored and any remaining tinnitus is usually masked by the increased volume of external sound heard by the patient.[1, p2403]

But Baloh disagrees, stating that in patients with otosclerosis whose chief compliant is tinnitus, the tinnitus frequently worsens despite a successful stapedectomy; If the stapedectomy is unsuccessful, the tinnitus often becomes unbearable.

Baloh continues: surgical treatment of tinnitus has generally been disappointing. Even patients who have undergone removal of acoustic neuromas report variable changes in their tinnitus. Of 500 patients who had acoustic neuromas removed, 83 percent had tinnitus before surgery: (tinnitus was the initial symptom in 11 percent): only 40 percent reported improvement. But 50 percent said their tinnitus was worse, and 10 percent had no change.[101, p17]

House and Brackmann gave a report of 29 patients who suffered from tinnitus and underwent cochlear implants. A cochlear implant is an electronic device assigned to generate electric stimulation of various segments of the cochlear branch of the cranial nerve. The implanted electronics are an induction coil which is imbedded in the bone inside the ear, an active electrode which is set in the middle ear, and a ground electrode which is placed in the eustachian tube area.

The external electronics include a microphone that is held at ear level by a hearing aid mould. The output of the microphone is fed to the stimulator, which is about the size of a body-type hearing aid. An electric current is transferred into the cochlea where the remaining cochlear neurons are excited to produce a sensation of sound.

Most patients with cochlear implants use their stimulators for 4-12 hours during their waking hours.

Eight patients reported that the tinnitus was absent, 15 said it was reduced, and six felt that it was the same. None of the patients reported tinnitus to be worse after use of the implant.[83, pp209-210]

An article in the ATA Newsletter reveals that for deaf patients, a cochlear implant may be appropriate. (The deaf also can suffer from tinnitus.)[7i]

TOPICAL APPLICATION TO THE EAR CANAL

Of all the attempts I made to relieve my tinnitus, overnight flooding of the outer ear canal with onion juice was the first one that was significantly effective. I first made the juice in my Champion juicer (available in health food stores). I put half an eyedropperful-no more-in the ringing ear. With more than that, the insertion of cotton to prevent the juice from running out would apply too much pressure on the ear drum.

I did that at bedtime, and when I awoke the next morning the ringing was gone! I thought I was rid of it for good, but after two days the tinnitus was back again. I warmed up the bottle of leftover onion juice in a cup of hot water and tried it again. It puzzled me that this time there was no effect.

Later I realized that the first onion juice I used was freshly made. A fresh onion will make your eyes tear when peeling it, but an old refrigerated onion won't-or at least it causes less tearing. The ingredient that causes the eyes to tear apparently is the one that relieved my tinnitus. So I made fresh onion juice, this time in a garlic press. A tablespoon of chopped onion produces enough juice.

Again I experienced several days of relief, but the tinnitus ultimately returned. I decided not to continue using the onion juice because the delicate membranes of the ear canal could not take the continuous abuse of such an irritating substance.

When I read Carmen's book, he stated that ear drops are prescribed for certain conditions of the outer or middle ear, and do not affect, nor are intended to affect the inner ear. Ear drops cannot restore hearing in cases of neural damage. They can help in treatment of itching, discomfort, or infection. Most importantly, ear drops should only be used upon the recommendation of your physician.[12, p70]

Swiss Labs, Inc.* offers herbal ear drops for temporary relief of tinnitus (2 to 4 hours). Their brochure states that the drops "will relieve ringing, buzzing, and pain in the ears by stimulating the blood supply to the nerves. Though not a cure...used regularly over a period of time, the drops will offer unquestionable relief, if not eliminate symptoms completely."

Another company, Health Fest*, offers herbal ear drops making the same claim as Swiss Labs, Inc. Their product's name is ProZaine E, and it contains aloe vera.

I tried many of the experiments that went into this book, and several of them gave me only partial relief. It seemed that there was something in my body more powerful than any remedy I had tried.

ULTRASOUND IRRADIATION

An issue of the American Tinnitus Association newsletter reported that Bihari and his coworkers in Japan had accidentally discovered that low-powered ultrasound relieved tinnitus in a patient being treated for other problems. This accidental finding led them to conduct an ultrasound study on 40 tinnitus patients where the low-powered ultrasound was applied to the ear. Only 28 patients completed the study but all 28 experienced relief of tinnitus as compared to placebo trials. The patient can neither hear nor feel the ultrasound, making placebo use viable.

Jack Vernon, Ph.D., who wrote the article, expressed his concern that the investigators had made no mention of possible damage to hearing; he suggested constant checks of high-frequency effects on their patients during treatment.[7j]

There is a difference between "low-powered" ultrasound and industrial airborne ultrasound.

W. I. Acton, from the Wolfson Unit for Noise and Vibration Control reported that although there is no evidence of permanent biological changes, including hearing loss, as a result of normal industrial exposures to pure ultrasound, some effects may occur as a result of experimental laboratory exposures. (This report is dated December, 1974.) But high levels of high-frequency audible sound which accompany many industrial processes may cause headaches, nausea, tinnitus, and possibly fatigue in persons without hearing loss at those frequencies.

Ultrasonic devices are widely used in production industries for a variety of operations, among them drilling, dicing, soldering, cleaning, welding plastics, emulsification, mixing liquids, etc.

When jet aircraft were introduced, the term "ultrasonic sickness" was coined to cover many diverse symptoms which included excessive fatigue, headache, nausea, vomiting, a loss of the sense of equilibrium, dizziness, etc., experienced by personnel working in their vicinity. Jet aircraft can produce high-frequency audible sounds between 160 and 165 dB. Control of ultrasound has been achieved by using conventional ear protectors.[94]

For anyone who is particularly interested in this subject, there is a later, but similar report dated 1983.[104, 105]

YOGA EXERCISES

Increasing circulation of blood to the head has been reported to alleviate tinnitus symptoms. The following yoga exercises may help:

- Sit in a comfortable position.
- Turn your head slowly to the right as far as it will comfortably go--keeping your chin tucked in. Hold this position for a few seconds. Then turn your head slowly to the left as far as it will comfortably go, again keeping your chin tucked in. Hold for a few seconds.
- Repeat 3 times.
- Tilting your head forward, bring your chin toward your chest and hold for a few seconds. Then tilt your head backward while keeping your chin tucked in and return to the starting position.
- Repeat 3 times.

PSYCHOLOGICAL INTERVENTION

BIOFEEDBACK

Richard Carmen, MD, of Glendale, California, and Dion Svihovec, MD, at the Veterans Administration Hospital in Sepulveda, California, affirmed that stress is a major contributor to biological degeneration, including deterioration of the cochlear system. Tinnitus and sensorineural hearing loss are often symptomatic of the constriction of nerves.

They have found electromyographic (EMG) biofeedback effective in the treatment of tinnitus. The instrumentation monitors muscle activity and presents the patient with auditory or visual signals representing that activity. The purpose of this procedure is to make it possible for the patient to gain a measure of voluntary control of involuntary processes.

With the aid of EMG feedback, tinnitus sufferers can learn to reduce or eliminate their annoyance reaction to tinnitus. The tinnitus patient listens to clicks reflecting moment-to-moment muscle tension for 20-30 minutes and somehow learns to reduce the auditory clicks, evidence that he has been able to relax the target muscle. Listening with eyes closed in a quiet room, perhaps reclining, seems ideal for inducing relaxation.

Carmen and Svihovec also found that if the EMG biofeedback treatment is not available or not desired, you may be able to by-pass the need for an external feedback device through the use of your own biological feedback system-if you are willing and sensitive enough, and if you can find a therapist able to properly direct at least the initial sessions.

They say that one excellent technique for the relaxation approach is listening to one's own breathing, listening to the flow and rhythm of each breath, slowing the breathing down progressively while realizing that the longer the pause between breaths, the greater the relaxation. As a result, the patient can use breath rate as feedback to monitor tension. This allows patients to become their own relaxation therapists whenever needed.

Relaxation is a state of mind and body during which muscle tension and mental activity are reduced. There are a wide range of relaxation processes available to treat tinnitus sufferers, from a rigid procedure such as progressive relaxation (alternately tensing and relaxing a series of muscles) to effective procedures such as listening to soft, flowing music or sound effects like falling rain, ocean waves, and wind.

Carmen and Svihovec have provided a program of seven audio cassettes for self-help, called "Eliminating the Annoyance of Ringing in the Ears, 1984." It is available from Auditory Research*[106]

HOLISTIC THERAPY

Paul Yanick, Jr., PhD, in private practice at the Woodbridge Hearing Center in Woodbridge, NJ, believes that biofeedback and other relaxation techniques are useful in reducing tension and helping the patient successfully adapt to stress. But he also feels that in order to achieve optimum results, such techniques should be combined with improvements in diet, nutrition, and exercise.

Yanick makes the following observations. Often the association of the ear as an integral part of the entire body seems to be disregarded, even though the biochemical bases of disease

130

and dysfunction present no more fundamental differences in the ear than elsewhere in the body. The sensory cells of the inner ear are like all living cells in our bodies in needing not only water, oxygen, and a suitable surrounding temperature, but a combination of over 40 nutrients all blended in the right proportions and working together.

Yanick theorizes that inadequate diet and nutrient intake, lack of exercise, and environmental stress factors may affect the genetically weakened ear in one or more of the following ways:

1. Inadequate blood flow via the small vessels feeding the cells of the inner ear usually results from the body's response to stress. The stress-fighting adrenal glands respond to stress by secreting various hormones, of which adrenaline is almost entirely responsible for the constriction of the small vessels of the inner ear in some individuals.

2. Excess toxic wastes and poor nutrition delivery via the blood vessels can destroy the strength and permeability of the capillaries. These toxins build up from an excessive use of aspirin and other drugs, quinine, smoking and dietary chemical poisons. It is from the capillaries that the cells of the inner ear receive the oxygen and nutrients from the bloodstream.

3. Imbalance between the sodium and potassium electrolytes can be triggered by the adrenal gland during its response to stress.

4. Diminished oxygen due to inadequate exercise and/or one of the above mentioned conditions can reduce energy production by the oxygen-dependent cells in the inner ear.

5. Diminished glucose supply to the cell environment of the inner ear can be caused by hypoglycemia and/or any

one of the above malfunctions. The inner ear has the highest energy requirements of any organ in the body. Glucose is the chief energy source for the ear.

6. An excess of nutrients (as in synthetic vitamins and minerals) can be expected to upset the metabolic rate and/or delicate biochemical balances of the hearing organ.

7. The most common causes of tinnitus are lymph and liver toxicity, biochemical imbalances caused by diet, drugs, stress, and digestive disorders. (See information about my book on indigestion at the end of this book.) Long-term consumption of acid food decreases the body's energy and suppresses immunity, while long-term ingestion of alkaline foods nourishes and revitalizes.[107]

In a book review of Yanick's latest book, Natural Relief from Tinnitus, in Health News & Review, he talks about his own battle with tinnitus which began as a teenager. His body was very acidic from eating too much animal protein and from the prescription drugs he took for asthma and allergies. (Yanick states that the pH (acid or alkaline balance) was acidic in all of his patients with ear disorders and the acid pH suppressed enzyme activity, causing the enzymatic complexes of mineral elements to become electrically unstable.) He began to measure his salivary and urine pH based on different diets. (Use phenaphtazine paper, available in drug stores.) A diet high in animal protein and low in carbohydrates and vegetables showed high acidic pH reading.

His experimentation with a vegetarian diet brought on a very slow, but progressive improvement in his pH. But actual improvements in his hearing and tinnitus did not improve until he stopped the megavitamins and replaced them with whole food supplements like spirulina, green barley, organic pumpkin seed oil or raw seeds, fresh ginger root, and fresh, raw carrot juice.

Yanick advises the reader not to expect immedite improvements on this program. Usually, the process of correcting long-term deficiency states and biochemical imbalances will take months.

Although I disagree with his excessive use of suplements which stresses the body by forcing it to digest and assimilate unnatural foods, I highly recommend this book.

Listed on "Books" in RESOURCE section.

SELF-REGULATION

Lawrence P. Ince, PhD, of the Department of Rehabilitation Medicine at Goldwater Memorial Hospital, New York City, tried a self-regulating approach for his tinnitus patients. They were seated in a sound chamber, and given headphones, and asked to describe their tinnitus symptoms in terms of frequency, loudness, and type of sound. The sound they described was duplicated by a synthesizer and played back to them at a level 5 dB softer than their own tinnitus.

"We matched our sound to their tinnitus," Ince reports. "Then we lowered our sound and asked patients to concentrate on lowering theirs. Each time they matched it, we lowered ours another 5 dB and just kept going. Eventually we came down the scale until their tinnitus was near or below their hearing threshold." One patient reduced her tinnitus by 34 dB. Follow-up showed her tinnitus was no longer a problem.[90, Sept. 1984, pp153-154]

VERBAL THERAPY

One Sunday afternoon a friend of mine came to visit. I have a very high regard for this man because of his high intelligence and his success in the business world. He was quite anxious to tell me about a method of stopping one's tinnitus by making a certain sound. He heard this on a tape he was listening to titled, "Magical Mind, Magical Body," by Dr. Deepak Chopra, an endocrinologist.[108] Chopra believes that the mind is not only in your brain but in every cell of the body, and by changing your thoughts about your body, you actually make your body itself change.

My friend said the sound was the letter "n." It must be said in a continuous sound, like "ennnnnnnn," for as long as your breath holds out. Do it about three times a day.

I thanked my friend politely, but was amazed that a man of his intellect would pass on such nonsense.

Monday passed and I thought about the "n" word but didn't practice the method.

On Tuesday I recalled that I use the sound "ohm" with good results for sleeping and relaxation. The sound "ohm" is a Hindu sacred word (a mantra) used repetitiously. "Ohm" is a "body sound," and "n" is a "mind sound." Perhaps the "n" word creates a particular vibration in the ear that "balances" the internal organs of the ear. I tried it three times and nothing happened. On Wednesday I tried it again and by the time I got to the 10th "n" sound, I felt my head get full of air and my left ear (where the tinnitus is) popped. I felt an immediate reduction in the intensity of the tinnitus.

Others have tried it with the same positive results. No one in the group had tinnitus as a result of trauma, so I would be very interested in knowing if this mantra has helped anyone if their tinnitus is the result of noise or physical trauma. I recommend the set of six audio cassettes very highly.

ALIMENTARY INTERVENTION

This section concerns changes we can make in what we put in or take out of our digestive tube, which runs through our bodies from the mouth to the anus.

DRUGS

My medical doctor diagnosed by tinnitus as "congestion of the inner ear combined with a retracted negative pressure." He also suggested I take a prescription drug named Entex LA (phenylpro-panolamine hydrochloride/guaifenesin). After reading the contraindications, I returned it to the pharmacist. Here are some of the warnings: Should be used with caution in patients with hypertension, diabetes mellitus, heart disease, peripheral vascular disease, hyper- thyroidism, or prostatic hypertrophy. I felt the toxic side effects would be worse than the tinnitus.

Abraham Shulman, MD, reports on a clinical study of 38 patients given antihistamine to reduce or eliminate tinnitus. A complete evaluation is essential to find patients amenable to treatment. Clinicians found that 22 patients with middle ear inflammation and eustachian tube dysfunction received total relief from antihistamine therapy. But, Shulman warns, prolonged treatment is necessary to get relief, and it must be kept in mind not only that antihistamines can produce a stimulating or depressing effect, but such effects can be additive.[115]

Durk Pearson and Sandy Shaw tell of Sandy's hearing and tinnitus being cured with Hydergine. Sandy's hearing suffered severe damage as a result of 6600 rads of radiation through her aural-oral region following the removal of a malignant salivary gland (parotid) tumor. Severe tinnitus developed in both ears, and her ability to hear high frequencies was severely damaged.

Sandy began using Hydergine. At first, using 3 to 6 milligrams of Hydergine per day for several months, Sandy didn't notice any changes in her hearing. She then increased her dosage to 12 milligrams per day in response to a scientific report she had read. In a few weeks, she began to notice small sounds, especially high frequency ones, that she hadn't noticed before. Then the level of her tinnitus began to decrease. She is now using 20 milligrams of Hydergine daily, looking for possible further improvements.[116]

One of the most promising, yet preliminary, studies suggests that terfenadine -- the common allergy drug commercially called Seldane -- may partially or completely relieve tinnitus. Ronald G. Amedee, M.D., assistant professor of otolaryngology at Tulane Medical Center, gave 24 tinnitus patients a 60 milligram tablet twice a day for three 30-day periods. Seventeen of the 24 showed some improvement in their tinnitus.[117]

Jack Vernon did a double-blind, placebo-controlled study in which 76% of patients on Xanax got relief from their tinnitus. Relief was defined as a reduction in the loudness of tinnitus by 40% or more. One side effect of Xanax is that it makes most patients drowsy. In the study, no patient obtained relief in the first week, and only a few in the next three weeks. Most patients did not experience relief until 5 to 9 weeks.[118]

In a double-blind controlled trial in nine patients with tinnitus, Dr's den Hartigh and C.G. Hilders* gave intravenous administration of lidocaine plasma to nine patients. No patient showed any effect during the placebo infusion. Administratin of lidocaine resulted in total suppression or suppression to a non-annoying level of tinnitus in five patients, slight suppression but still annoying tinnitus in two patients, and worsening tinnitus in one patient. No effect of lidocaine was observed in one patient. Notable side effects were observed if the dosage was too high.

*The department of Clinical Pharmacy, University Medical Centre, Leiden, The Netherlands. Clin Pharmaco Ther 1993 Oct;54(4):415-20.

Note: Be sure to check, at the end of this chapter, the list of over 100 prescription drugs that cause tinnitus. This information was taken from the 1993 PDR GUIDE TO DRUG INTERACTIONS, SIDE EFFECTS, & INDICATIONS. SIDE EFFECTS INDEX, pgs 1228-1229. I received a call recently from a woman in New York who complained to her doctor about her sudden onset of tinnitus. Two of the drugs he prescribed were actually on this list!

HERBS, VITAMINS AND MINERALS

The American Tinnitus Association newsletter tells of a clinic in West Germany that used ginkgo biloba on 64 patients with inner ear or nerve deafness. The clinic reported that the herb improved damaged hearing nerves, and that in most cases the tinnitus was eliminated. Ginkgo biloba is a highly purified extract obtained from the dried leaves of the ginkgo biloba tree. The active ingredients in the extract supposedly have an effect on cell metabolism, increasing glucose consumption in areas where there is a poor blood supply.[7k]

The clinical testing was uncontrolled, meaning that the tree extract was not compared with an inactive substance or placebo. Only half the group was experiencing tinnitus: 30 percent of these said their tinnitus disappeared but 50 percent reported no change in their symptoms.

Ginkgo Biloba is available at health food stores.

An article in The American Journal of Otology by George S. Shambaugh Jr, MD, reports the possibility of using zinc for the control of tinnitus. Chemical analysis of the zinc content of sensory tissues in the cochlea shows the highest level of zinc in any organ or tissue in the body. Shambaugh proposes that tissues and organs especially high in an essential trace element may suffer structural and functional impairment from its deficiency. Zinc deficiency increases after age 60, and may be a factor in some cases of presbycusis, tinnitus, and imbalance.[119]

After the first edition of my book was out, I received a letter from a woman in Germany. She told me about a book titled Health Through God's Pharmacy, published by Wilhelm Ennsthaler in Steyr, Austria. The book recommends Swedish bitters for hearing loss. She claimed that the remedy reduced the degree of her tinnitus. Swedish bitters can be found in many health food stores. Nature Works Incorporated, in Agoura HIlls, California, is the distributor for the German maker of this product.

Fenugreek seeds helped Leota Lane of Eugene, Oregon*, rid herself of "cricket" noises in her ears. She puts 2 ½ full soup spoons of fenugreek seeds in 3 cups of cold water and lets it set overnight. The following morning she stirs the mixture a little, separates the liquid from the seeds, then drinks the liquid. Then she immediately pours another cup of water on top of the seeds so that another mixture will be ready to drink later in the evening. She follows that twice-a-day routine for several days until the seeds have lost their strength. If you prefer warm tea, heat the liquid after you separate it from the seeds: heating the seeds will make the tea too bitter to drink.

*Heineiman's Encyclopedia of Fruits, Vegetables & Herbs, Parker Publishing Co., N.Y., 1988.

Another herbal remedy is included in the same book for tinnitus using the empty shell of sunflower seeds.

Bring 1 ½ pints of water to a boil. Add 2 tbsps. Each of crushed seeds and their empty shells. Cover, reduce heat and simmer for 15 minutes. Remove from heat and steep an additional half hour. Drink 1 cup of lukewarm tea, after straining, every 4 to 6 hours.

Linda Rector-Page suggests a program for tinnitus in her book, Healthy Healing:

> 1. Go on a short 3-day mucous cleansing diet. Then eat fresh foods for the rest of the week. Have plenty of salads and citrus fruits.
> 2. For a month, eat a mildly cleansing diet. Avoid all clogging, saturated fat foods. Reduce dairy products. Add plenty of fiber foods from vegetables and whole grains.
> 3. Drink only [distilled] bottled water.
> 4. Have a glass of lemon juice and water each morning.
> 5. Keep the diet very low in sugars, salt and dairy foods.
> 6. Take licorice root extract.
> 7. Drink summer savory and rose water tea. They

can also be used as ear drops.

JUICING

The book <u>Juicing for Life</u> offers juice recipes specifically for tinnitus.

Apple Shake

1/2 orange, peeled (leave white pithy part)
2 green apples, seeded
1 ripe banana
1 Tbsp. brewer's yeast
Orange slice for garnish

Juice orange and apple. Place juice, banana, and yeast in blender or food processor, and blend until smooth. Garnish with orange slice.

Beneficial Juices:

Beet -- a potent detoxifier.
Kale and parsley -- sources of iron.
Spinach, kale, beet green, and sweet pepper -- sources of folic
 acid.
Green pepper and apple -- sources of chromium.
Spinach, turnip greens, and beet greens -- sources of
 manganese.
Green bean -- source of choline.[120]

REDUCING WEIGHT

I have included this chapter for those who must reduce weight due to high blood pressure, and for those using diuretics as part of a weight reducing program. Also, the many problems associated with obesity prompt use of the pharmaceutical industry's plethora of drugs contributing to our internal load of toxins.

T. C. Fry claims that none of the "miracle diet pills" on the market have helped the more than 82 million overweight Americans lose excess pounds permanently. The facts concerning "diet pills" are so shocking that even the AMA's latest guide to medicine does not recommend most of them as an aid to weight loss. They are also largely ineffective due to the fact that once the individual goes off the pills, not only is his body chemistry upset, but also his body is further devitalized and weakened by the poison in the pills. Add to those facts a lack of proper nutrition while dieting, and the body's craving for nutrients, and the dieter has an even harder time keeping from overeating.[25t]

Shelton explains that since obesity results from habitually eating more food than is used by the body in its activities, in combination with a diet consisting of a high percentage of animal fats and processed foods usually high in fat, it becomes obvious that weight can be reduced not only by eating less each day than is required by the body, but by eating proportionally more fruits and vegetables, preferably in their raw state.[25u] (The significance of raw food will be covered in the next chapter.)

The best procedure in losing weight and keeping it off is to rid the body of toxins and eat moderate amounts of the proper foods. Fasting has proved to be the quickest, easiest, and most satisfactory means of reducing weight. (Fasting is covered in more depth in the next chapter.) Strict discipline must be maintained after the fast so as not to regress to old eating habits.

Severen L. Schaeffer is the director of a center in France whose members eat only raw food. He explains why people

141

become overweight when they eat cooked foods.

When food is eaten in its original state, and when the body has had been replenished in the nutrients that particular food has to offer, it no longer wants more. Body chemistry changes our appetite for that food, and the taste becomes unpleasant even though the eater may still be hungry. But this mechanism functions only with foods that have not been denatured in any way, and only when eaten in isolation-that is, when it's unmixed with other foods and unseasoned.

This phenomenon does not occur with foods that have been frozen, cooked, chopped, ground, etc., or with extracts such as juices or oils. Cooking food alters its original molecular structure, to which we are genetically adapted. Once cooked, it will taste good and continue to do so indefinitely because its thermally modified structure will not trigger a taste-change response. As a consequence, we can continue to eat it with un-diminished pleasure until we're full, ingesting many times the amount we require.[121]

Shelton continues: exercise is another way to lose weight, but the amount of exercise required is extremely time consuming. To lose two pounds of fat would require walking 104 miles or sawing wood for 10 hours straight. These comparisons show how little food you actually use in doing work and the fallacy of the belief that to do heavy work one must eat great quantities of food. This does not, however, mean that one should not exercise. Exercise is imperative for the maintenance of muscle tone while reducing.

Exercise must be coupled with dietary control for successful weight reduction. It is necessary for one to reduce the amount of food eaten, as well as to carefully select the food, if one is to lose weight. Fresh fruits such as oranges, grapefruits, tangerines, pineapples, and apples, and all fresh raw green vegetables are the best foods on which to reduce.

Any person reducing and weighing daily is sure to be disappointed and discouraged. No reducing program will produce consistent day-to-day changes. At first you reduce quite rapidly, then the rate of loss slows down after the first two or three weeks. Much determination is required to successfully reduce when one is overweight, and the very love of eating and indifference to personal appearance that permitted the original gain in weight are the chief obstacles to persistent and consistent effort.

I have never had an overweight problem but nevertheless because of my allergies and tendency toward chronic fatigue, I had to eventually omit everything in my diet except fresh fruit and vegetables (even nuts because of their rancidity). I would like to share a mathematical mental exercise I used to help me through the withdrawal of eliminating bread, meat, milk, eggs, butter, pasta and cooked food.

My basic symptoms from eating these foods were insomnia, foggy thinking, diarrhea, and chronic fatigue, which prevented me from functioning to my fullest ability. I calculated thusly; of the 24 hours in a day I sleep an average of eight of those hours, leaving 16 waking hours. To round the figures out, let's say it takes one hour to eat meals. That leaves 15 hours to do whatever activities I pursue, which give meaning to life. I chose not to sacrifice those 15 hours for the one hour of enjoyment I got from eating forbidden foods.

I sincerely hope this "mathematical psychology" is helpful.

RAW/LIVE FOOD AND FASTING

This chapter tells of my success in freeing myself of tinnitus. I have tried many of the therapies in this book with no permanent success. Four members of the group also went on

143

a raw food diet and a fast. They were also successful in stopping their tinnitus.

I realize that the concept of eating raw food may be totally foreign to the reader, so allow me to give you the essential, fundamental facts.

For over a million years our ancestors ate food basically as they found it in nature. They did not elaborately prepare food-they were savages. Today's man evolved from eating food in the condition as it was found in nature.

You are what you eat, and those of our ancestors who were most accurate in selecting their food were the healthiest and produced the most offspring. Those who made poor choices in selecting their food tended to die sooner.[122]

Schaeffer expands on this thought: to give you a graphic picture of the importance of eating raw food, imagine the course of evolution as a road 25 miles long. Men would be coming into existence only 70 yards from the end. The discovery of cooking happened 25 feet from the end. The development of agriculture arrived about five inches before our time.

For nearly the whole length of this road, our predecessors ate only what they could find or catch. Their instinct selected the food by smell and taste. The process of natural selection ensures survival only for species that are adapted to their environments. In biochemical terms, the survivors would be those whose DNA programmed them organismically to detect, select, ingest, digest, and metabolize the kinds of available foods they needed to survive.

Given the time-span involved in evolutionary processes, has man had time to become genetically adapted to foodstuffs that have been progressively transforming since he started

144

using fire? Even though man has undertaken omnivorous eating practices, our anatomy and physiology have not changed.

Susan Hazard, PhD, further explains in an article titled, "What's Wrong with Cooked Food," that Homosapiens is the only species on earth that eats cooked foods, and the only species of the entire animal kingdom that is sick (except for domesticated animals that eat what we feed them). The high application of heat destroys vitamins and minerals. Vitamin A and E are oxidized and destroyed. Vitamin C and all members of the vitamin B complex are water soluble, therefore easily destroyed. Not only are these vitamins destroyed, but their residue is unusable and toxic when ingested.

Minerals are required to sustain the alkalinity of body fluids; they are essential for structure, in healing and repair. Cooking fragments food because it disrupts the mineral organization, rendering it inorganic, unusable and toxic.

Heating any food above approximately 122 degrees Fahrenheit destroys the food enzymes. Enzymes are essential triggers in metabolic activity of all living things. Even though humans have the ability to manufacture their own cellular enzymes from nutrients, this requires raw foods to support the body's own enzyme system. Within each food are those enzymes needed to properly digest and assimilate it. When we destroy enzymes in food through cooking, our body has to make more of its own digestive enzymes to properly digest and assimilate food. But as we age our body's enzyme-producing abilities tend to wane. Adjustment by the body to the eating of cooked, enzyme-poor food is always done at the expense of vitality, endurance and strength.

Cooking food chemically changes protein molecules, making them toxic and less digestible. The vital factors in

145

protein, the amino acids, are destroyed and rendered useless, thereby making it impossible for the human body to build its own protein from food. And because the molecular structures are altered, they are more subject to putrefaction in the intestines.

Cooking fat-containing foods renders the fat and the foods less digestible and highly toxic, and has been shown to be carcinogenic in experiments on animals.

Starches are subject to fermentation and are transformed into toxic wastes by cooking. Acetic acid (vinegar) is formed, stimulating the thyroid gland, and leaching out the body's phosphorus which is essential for adrenal gland performance. Eventually, both the thyroid and adrenal start to dysfunction.

People who primarily depend on cooked starches often experience headaches, throat congestion, mucous expectoration, pains in the heart, body odor, frequent chills, and rapid pulse.[25v]

I conclude: cooked food is not assimilated, no nourishment is gained, the undigested food becomes toxic in the body, enervation sets in, then disease, and finally death. Raw food prevents the degeneration of the body and promotes health.

The eating of raw food is the result of science of natural hygiene. Natural hygiene is a school of thought in which diseases are held to be caused by improper life practices, especially dietary indiscretions. Illness is felt to stem from toxicosis as the result of internally generated wastes, from ingested substances, or both. It is brought on by dissipation, stress, overindulgence, excess or deficiency of the normal essentials of life, and pollution of the body with substances not normal to it. Accordingly, recovery from sickness can be achieved only by discontinuing its causes and supplying conditions favorable to healing.[25w]

Marti Fry, asserted that fasting is the fastest way to regain health. Abstinence from all food for a period of time allows the body to redirect its energies from the tasks of digestion and assimilation to the task of purification and repair. However, it must always be kept in mind that the fast is only the beginning. You cannot fast, become completely well, and then indulge in unhealthful living and eating practices, or you will become more sick.

Before you begin a fast, decide on a daily exercise program, learn which foods are beneficial to the body and which are harmful, learn how to correctly combine your foods for best digestion, learn to eat in moderation, and understand that you must take sufficient time to rest and relax. Specifically, learn how to live healthfully. Give up all the disease-causing factors such as smoking, drinking, junk or sugared foods, salt and other condiments, laziness, staying up late at night, and overeating. Then you will be ready for a fast.

Most people will have to undergo more than one fast to rid their bodies of the accumulation of toxins from a lifetime of abusing the body.

You can fast during your regular vacation or a three-day weekend; you won't be losing anything but your toxins. Fasting is an investment in your health and future.[25x]

In a response to an inquirer, T. C. Fry tells of his own experience with tinnitus that developed when he had malaria and was injected with quinine. His body deposited much of the drug around the cochlea and otic nerves. The reaction of the tissue and nerves in the area in trying to shake free this toxic substance was just the reverse of their normal hearing functions. Instead of receiving and translating external vibrations into sound, the tissues vibrated and transmitted their own sound.

He explains that almost any drug or toxic material can do this-even the body's own waste materials. Thus, the same cause for all of our diseases: body toxicity. He continues, in response to the inquirer's question about a masker: T o try to mask tinnitus with sounds that drown out the ringing, humming, or crackling is on the same order as butting your head against a concrete wall to drown out a headache.

Get down to basics and find out what causes the problem. Knowing that toxicity causes the problem, we narrow it down to seeking causes of toxemia. One of the foremost sources for toxicity of the body is, of all things, cooked foods-something you've foresworn to keep in your diet. If eating cooked foods is more important to you than debility and suffering, then you've earned it.

Fry continues: people who suffer from tinnitus have the propensity to discharge toxins in the otic area. Other people's body make-up discharges their toxins in the form of acne, arthritis, headaches, herpes, etc. The body will clear up the tinnitus once the toxins are reduced below the point that the otic nerve is no longer irritated.

Exercise, fresh pure air, adequate rest and sleep, etc., are all essential to a body free of impairing toxicity. I suggest that you start out by going on a fast of at least seven days. Your humming should cease after the third or fourth day.

Remember, as long as the causes are continued, your problems will continue.[25y]

I was quite familiar with the many advantages of eating raw food, but whenever I tried to eat raw foods at a meal, I would experience extreme hunger and stomach discomfort, causing me to avoid them.

148

Later I learned why in reading Fry's response to a woman with the same problem. Fry explained that the woman's body had become accommodated to cooked foods. The symptoms of discomfort can be labeled withdrawal symptoms, and the best way to overcome them is to undertake a total withdrawal from foods for a while. This will enable the body to cleanse and repair itself. This should be done under supervision.

People whose bodies are very toxic experience "withdrawal" symptoms when they make a drastic change toward an improved diet. For example, when the use of a toxic stimulant such as coffee is stopped suddenly, headaches are common and a letdown occurs. This is due to the discard by the body of the toxins caffeine and theobromine, which are removed from the tissues and transported through the bloodstream to the eliminating organs. When the blood circulates through the brain during its many bodily rounds, these irritants register in our consciousness as pain. Other signs of the body's detoxifying are discomfort in the back, with its heavy concentration of nerve cells.

With an improved diet, remarkable things begin to happen to the body and mind. The amazing intelligence present in every cell of the body is stimulated. The rule may be stated thusly: when the quality of food coming into the body is of higher quality than the elements present in body tissues, the body begins to discard the lower-grade materials to make room for the superior materials it uses to make new and healthier tissue.[25z]

Therefore, the introduction of raw foods into the diet should be done slowly. Start by replacing one of your normal meals each day with a raw one. Or use one steamed vegetable (like cauliflower) in the dish, and complement it with grated raw vegetables. Gradually eliminate meat and processed foods from your diet until you reach a balance of about 75 percent raw and 25 percent cooked. At this point you will discover the benefits of raw food. Note: If you have an electric stove, it is not necessary to keep the heat on when steaming vegetables. The residue from the hot plate will keep the steaming water at a high enough heat to soften all vegetables except cauliflower in five minutes.

My body was so toxic that the eating of raw foods alone was too slow a process to eliminate my body of them; a fast was essential. I went to a retreat near Austin, Texas, for a supervised seven-day fast. By the fifth day the tinnitus was gone. That was eight years ago.

On occasion if I eat the wrong food or am exposed to something to which I am sensitive, the tinnitus will flare up again-but at a barely noticeable level. At those times I prepare and drink fresh fruit or vegetable juices for one day, and by the next day the tinnitus goes away. I also use the "n" mantra. I now view the onset of tinnitus as a beneficial message that I've eaten a harmful food, and I omit it from my diet.

The side benefits of this diet are numerous. I have more energy, I require less sleep, I look younger, I'm more mentally alert, and I can deal with stress more readily. Plus, since I'm no longer spending hours in the kitchen cooking, washing greasy dishes and pots, and keeping the kitchen clean, I have more time to work on constructive projects.

In my search for exciting raw fruit and vegetable dishes, I was unable to find a recipe book that made raw food interesting. So I did a lot of experimenting and ended up writing my own recipe book. You will find information about my book, and an order sheet at the end of this book.

I hope for the sake of your overall health that you try eating more raw fruits and vegetables. Please pass the results on to me. I am interested in finding out about your tinnitus and what you may have done to restore and maintain good health. Also, it will enable me to expand the next edition with new information.

Note: Since writing my first edition of this book, I have written two recipe books: The Garden of Eden Raw Fruit & Vegetable Recipes which applies the dietary recommendations in this book, and The 10-Minute Vegetarian Cook Book which is a "transition" recipe book to acclimate your body to raw foods. I also wrote a book for those who frequently have indigestion: Stop Your Indigestion: Causes, Remedies and Recipes.

The order sheets are at the end of this book.

NEW INFORMATION

I have read in Howard Long's book, "TINNITUS and OTHER HEARING PROBLEMS," that he suggests using niacin, then lying on a slant board. One reader said he felt an improvement in two days.

It is very difficult to find slant boards. But I have found one called BODYSLANT. It is safer and easier to use than a regular slant board. It is also reasonably priced. Please see the information on the BODYSLANT in the back of the book.

ADDENDUM

TMJ and CRANIAL OSTEOPATHY

In an article written by Jack Alpan, D.D.S. and Toby Chamberlain, in Total Health Magazine,* they explain the importance of balance in curing TMJ Syndrome.

They discuss their experience with Mrs. B who developed TMJ after she had new dentures made. After studying her uneven features it was obvious that her entire head had been out of balance for many years, probably long before she graduated to dentures. As each tooth was lost and the empty space not filled by a replacement, surrounding teeth began to drift and an uneven bite developed, causing an imbalance in the jaw joint.

When all her teeth were gone and dentures made to fit the existing structure, without first correcting the jaw imbalance, the TMJ problem was compounded at an accelerated rate. While these changes were going on in her mouth, the bones in her head began to shift in order to balance out the jaw imbalance, which led to the TMJ Syndrome.

The doctors helped Mrs. B. By having her bite down on soft wax, which gave her temporary relief. Permanent relief was achieved by using a TENS (transcutaneous electro-neuromuscular stimulator) device and craniopathy therapy.

*For a copy of Doctor, This Pain is Killing Me!, send a business-sized, stamped, self-addressed envelope to:

Jack Alpan, D.D.S.
2440 W. Third Street
Los Angeles, CA 90057
(213) 383-3833

APPLIED KINESIOLOGY
& FOOD TESTING

You can test yourself for food allergies simply by asking the innate intelligence of the body. Stand with your feet slightly apart. Hold the food in your hands (OK to have it in a jar) close to your body. Close your eyes and continually ask yourself, "Is this good for me?" Soon your body will tilt forwards or backwards. If it tilts forward, it is fairly safe to eat (a 90% accuracy rate). If your body tilts backward, you can be certain you are allergic to it. If there is no movement with your body, the food is neither good nor bad, but I have seen cases where people were unable to get in touch with their inner self.

This test is also effective for mouthwash, toothpaste, dental floss, liquor, cigarettes, prescription drugs and illicit drugs.

1993 PDR GUIDE TO
DRUG INTERACTIONS
SIDE EFFECTS, AND INDICATIONS
SIDE EFFECTS INDEX
pages 1228-1229
ISBN 1-56363-021-4

Your physician should <u>always</u> be consulted about questions
before any changes are made in your medication.
Page numbers listed refer to 1993 edition of PDR.

(▨ Described in PDR For Nonprescription Drugs)

(◉ Described in PDR For Ophthalmology)

Incidence data in parenthesis; ▲ 3% or more

Tinnitus

Accutane Capsules (Less than
1%).. 1960
Actifed with Codeine Cough Syrup.. 769
Adapin Capsules (Infrequent) 1346
Alferon N Injection (One patient) 1879
Altace Capsules (Less than 1%)...... 1112
Amicar Syrup, Tablets, and
Injection (Occasional) 1223
▲ Anafranil Capsules (4% to 6%) 671
▲ Anaprox and Anaprox DS Tablets
(3-9%)... 2391

▲ Anestacon Solution (Among most
common).. 2508
Ansaid Tablets (1-3%) 2431
Aralen Hydrochloride Injection (1
patient).. 2134
Aralen Phosphate Tablets (1
patient).. 2135
Arthritis Strength BC Powder........ ▨ 516
Asacol Delayed-Release Tablets 1868
Ascriptin A/D Caplets 1926
Regular Strength Ascriptin Tablets 1926
Asendin Tablets (Less than 1%)...... 1225
Atretol Tablets 666
Atrofen Tablets (Rare)...................... 667
Atrohist Plus Tablets 557
Azactam for Injection (Less than
1%)... 2353
Azo Gantanol Tablets........................ 1969
Azo Gantrisin Tablets........................ 1970
Azulfidine Tablets and EN-tabs
(Rare) 1184
BC Powder .... ▨ 517
Bactrim DS Tablets........................... 1973
Bactrim I.V. Infusion.......................... 1971
Bactrim 1973
Children's Bayer Chewable
Aspirin .... ▨ 724

Genuine Bayer Aspirin Tablets &
Caplets... ▨ 724
Maximum Bayer Aspirin Tablets
& Caplets.. ▨ 725
Bayer Plus Aspirin Tablets.............. ▨ 726
Therapy Bayer Enteric Aspirin
Caplets .... ▨ 728
▲ 8 Hour Bayer Timed-Release
Aspirin (Among mots frequent).... ▨ 726
Benadryl Capsules.............................. 1745
Benadryl Injection 1746
Biocadren Tablets (Less than 1%) 1480
Arthritis Strength Bufferin
Analgesic Caplets 761
Buprenex Injectable (Less than
1%)... 1895
BuSpar (Frequent) 1454
Cama Arthritis Pain Reliever........ ▨ 682
Capastat Sulfate Vials 1283
Carbocaine Hydrochloride Injection 2137
Cardene Capsules (Rare) 2393
Cardioquin Tablets 1882
Cardizem CD Capsules-180 mg.
240 mg and 300 mg (Less
than 1%)... 1368
Cardizem SR Capsules-60 mg, 90
mg and 120 mg (Less than
1%)... 1372
Cardizem Tablets-30 mg, 60 mg,
90 mg and 120 mg (Less
than 1%)... 1374
Cardura Tablets (1%)........................ 2031
Cartrol Tablets (Less common)....... 509
Children's Advil Suspension (Less
than 3%).. 2537
Cibalith-S.. 900
Cipro I.V. (1% or less)...................... 1636
Cipro I.V. Pharmacy Bulk Package
(Less than 1%)................................. 1639
Cipro Tablets (Less than 1%) 1633
Clinoril Tablets (Greater than 1%) 1483

154

155

TELEPHONE HEARING SCREENING TEST

In an effort to create better hearing health awareness, hospitals and hearing health clinics in a nationwide network are setting up information systems to provide accurate information on hearing problems and hearing protection programs. Today it is now possible to take a preliminary hearing screening test over the telephone.

Callers will receive a prerecorded message and be given a simple screening test. Take the test in a quiet environment, using a good quality phone, and call more than once to be sure you have heard all eight tones.

There are local numbers to call in most of the 50 states. To obtain the number nearest you, call

1-800-222-EARS (3277).

In Pennsylvania call

215-565-6114.

This information is available by mail by writing to:

Occupational Hearing Services
PO Box 1880
Media, PA 19063

GLOSSARY

- A -

ABSOLUTE THRESHOLD: The threshold, in decibels at a given frequency in the absence of other sounds.

ADDICTION: The state of devoting oneself habitually or compulsively to an activity or habit-forming substance, resulting in the inability to stop without experiencing pain or discomfort.

AFLATOXINS: Powerful toxins and carcinogens produced by molds and commonly found in growing crops, foods improperly harvested or stored, and in marijuana cigarettes. Crops commonly contaminated by aflatoxins are grains, legumes, nuts and seeds (especially peanuts).

AIR BONE GAP: Occurs when pure tones are heard more loudly through the bones behind the ear rather than through the eardrum. Indicates conductive hearing loss (a problem in the middle ear).

ALLERGEN: A substance that causes an allergic reaction.

ALLERGY: An abnormal response to a substance well tolerated by most people.

ANTIBIOTICS: The group of drugs usually prepared from molds or mold-like organisms, which are effective against bacteria but not viruses.

ANTIHISTAMINE: Any of certain drugs that neutralize the vasoconstrictor action of histamine in the body, used especially in the treatment of allergic conditions, as hay fever, asthma, etc., and of the common cold.

ANTIOXIDANT: A substance that slows down the process of oxidation; used for detoxification, it offers some protection against air pollution.

ANTIPYRETIC: Preventive or alleviative of fever. A medicine to allay fever.

AUDIOGRAM: A graph depicting absolute sound threshold or hearing level measured in the absence of other sounds.

AUDIOLOGIST: A nonmedical university-trained specialist who is qualified to evaluate hearing problems.

AUDITORY CANAL: The ear canal, a funnel-shaped hair-lined passage that contains wax-secreting glands.

AURAL: Pertaining to the ear or the sense of hearing.

AURICLE: The outer ear; passes sound waves to middle ear.

- B -

BONE CONDUCTOR HEARING AIDS: Used when the ear canal is closed or drainage is severed. Sounds are heard (rather poorly) through the bone behind the ear.

- C -

CALCIFICATION: The hardening of tissues through the deposition of calcium salts.

CANDIDA: A genus of yeast-like fungi normally found in the body but which can multiply and cause infections, allergic sensitivity or toxicity.

CARCINOGEN: A substance that causes cancer.

CAROTID: Of, pertaining to, or near one of the two major arteries on each side of the neck.

CERUMEN: Ear wax.

CERVICAL: Of, pertaining to, or near the neck, in the context used herein.

CHEMOTHERAPY: The use of drugs or medication in the treatment or control of disease.

COLONIC IRRIGATION: A deep enema purported to aid the body in expelling toxic materials.

COCHLEA: A snail-shaped, fluid-filled structure in the inner ear; controls balance and converts sound waves to nerve impulses.

COCHLEA IMPLANT: Implants intended to replace part or all of the inner ear.

CONDUCTIVE HEARING LOSS: Hearing loss due to abnormalities in the conductive apparatus of the ear, meaning the outer and middle ear.

- D -

DECIBEL: A measure of sound intensity.

DETOXIFICATION: The process of removing toxic (poisonous) substances from the body.

- E -

EARDRUM: A thin, flexible membrane separating the outer ear and middle ear.

ELECTRODE: Any terminal connecting a conventional conductor, as copper wire, with a non conventional one, as an electrolyte.

ENERVATE: To sap the strength of vitality of; weaken in body or will. Devitalized.

ENZYME: A protein produced by cells and having the power to initiate or accelerate specific chemical reactions in the metabolism of plants and animals.

EUSTACHIAN TUBE: A passage between the nasopharynx and the middle ear, serving to equalize air pressure between the tympanic cavity and the atmosphere.

- F -

FORMALDEHYDE: A colorless, pungent gas found in home building materials, automotive parts, plastics, textiles, embalming fluid, room deodorants, fungicides, cosmetics, and thousands of everyday products.

FREQUENCY (or pitch): Cycles per second (hertz).

- G -

GALVANIZE: To stimulate to muscular action by electricity.

GLYCEMIA: Sugar in the blood.

162

- H -

HAMMER: Middle ear bone.

HELIX: Margin of the external ear.

HERBALISM: The practice of treating illness with herbs.

HERTZ: Frequency, cycles per second.

HIGH FREQUENCY: As related to hearing; the upper part of the hearing range.

HOLISTIC: An approach to medicine that treats the person as a whole and focuses on prevention, nutrition, living habits, and a positive emotional outlook.

HOMEOPATHY: A branch of medicine based on the theory that a substance that produces symptoms in healthy persons will also, in minute doses, cure the same symptoms in diseased persons.

HORMONE: An internal secretion produced in and by one of the endocrine glands, as the pituitary, thyroid, adrenals, etc., and carried by the blood stream or body fluids to other parts of the body where it has a specific physiological effect.

HYPERGLYCEMIA: Excess blood sugar.

- I -

IMMUNE SYSTEM: The mechanism by which the body recognizes a material as foreign to itself and neutralizes, metabolizes, or eliminates it.

INTRACRANIAL: Occurring or situated within the cranium or skull.

IODINE: Chemical element once used as an antiseptic and therapeutic agent in medicine.

- J -

JUGULAR VEIN: Large vein at front of throat.

- L -

LABYRINTH: Internal ear.

LABYRINTHITIS: Inflammation of the labyrinth.

- M -

MANDIBULAR: Pertaining to the mandible or lower jaw bone.

MASKER: A device which introduces sounds into the ear in attempting to mask noises inside the head.

MASTOID: Bone situated behind the ear, nipple-shaped.

MASTOIDECTOMY: Surgical destruction of the cells in the mastoid.

MIDDLE EAR: The air-filled space between the eardrum and the inner ear. Contains the three smallest bones in the body.

164

- N -

NARCOTIC: Producing a state of unconsciousness; any sleep-inducing drug; one addicted to the use of narcotics.

NATURAL HYGIENE: A science which believes humans should live in harmony with nature, and that they are constitutionally adapted to a diet of fruit, vegetables, nuts, and seeds eaten in compatible combinations while in the fresh, raw, natural state. Natural hygienist also believe that disease is caused by improper life practices, especially dietary indiscretions, and that fasting is the most favorable condition under which an ailing body can purify and repair itself.

NATUROPATHY: A system of treating disease with nutrition, air, exercise and sunshine, and rejection of drug use.

NERVE LOSS (sensory-neural): A term to differentiate inner-ear problems from those in the middle ear (conductive hearing loss).

NEURITIS: Inflammation of a nerve.

NICOTINE: Poisonous alkaloid of tobacco.

NITRITES: Mainly used as a food and anti-bacterial preservative; nitrites are common in smoked meats such as bacon, hot dogs, and cold cuts. In the human digestive tract, they combine with other substances to form nitrosamines, which are carcinogenic.

- O -

ORGANIC FOODS: Foods grown without synthetic chemical fertilizers or the use of pesticides.

165

OTO: Combining form. Ear: pertaining to the ear.

OTOLARYNGOLOGY: The branch of medicine that treats of the ear and throat.

OTOSCLEROSIS: A type of conductive hearing loss caused when the tiny bones of the middle ear no longer transmit sound properly from the eardrum to the inner ear.

OTOLOGIST: A medical specialist in ear disease.

OTOTOXIC: Literally: poisonous to the ear. For example, some ototoxic drugs which may cause deafness are kanamycin, streptomycin, dihydrostreptomycin, aspirin, and quinine.

OUTGAS: To give off minute portions of chemical fumes from a solid substance.

OVAL WINDOW: The opening to the fluid-filled inner ear.

OXIDANT: A substance that promotes combination with oxygen to form new compounds.

- P -

PATHOLOGICAL: Related to, involving, concerned with, or caused by disease.

PENICILLIN: A powerful antibiotic found in the mold fungus penicillium and produced in several forms for the treatment of a wide variety of bacterial infections.

PETROCHEMICAL: A synthetic chemical derived from petroleum or natural gas.

PITCH: That attribute of sound described by frequency.

166

POLLUTANT: Any gaseous, chemical, or organic substance that contaminates water, the atmosphere or the physical body.

PRESBYCUSIS: A hereditary type of sensory-neural hearing loss that comes with aging.

PRESSURE: Stress; strain.

PROSTHESIS: The fitting of artificial parts to the body.

PURE TONE: A sound composed of only one frequency. Used in hearing tests.

- R -

RANCID: Having the unpleasant taste or smell of oily substances which have begun to spoil; rank; sour.

ROTATION DIET: A diet in which a particular food is eaten only once every five days.

- S -

SACRAL: Of, or pertaining to, or situated near the sacrum. A sacral vertebra or nerve.

SACRUM: A composite bone formed by the union of the five vertebrae between the lumbar and caudal regions (near the tail or posterior), constituting the dorsal part of the pelvis.

SENSORINEURAL HEARING LOSS: Hearing loss due to abnormalities in the sensory and neural elements of the auditory system.

SYNTHETIC: Man-made; not produced normally by nature.

- T -

TENSOR: Any muscle that extends or stretches a part of the body.

THRESHOLD: The minimum level at which a sound can be detected by a subject. (The criterion of detection is arbitrary, but should be specified.)

TOLERANCE THRESHOLD: The maximum amount of toxic substances a person can endure without reacting.

TONE DECAY: The tone becomes inaudible.

TOXEMIA: A condition resulting from the distribution of poisonous substances throughout the body.

TYMPANIC MEMBRANE: Another name for the eardrum.

- V -

VALSALVA MANEUVER: Forcible exhalation effort against a closed glottis. In more common terms it is performed by holding your nose and exhaling forcefully but gently.

VASOCONSTRICTOR: A nerve, drug, etc., causing constriction of a blood vessel.

VERTIGO: The illusion of movement of a person in relation to the environment. The patient feels that he himself is spinning (subjective type) or the objects are whirling about him (objective type).

VESTIBULE: Any of several chambers or channels adjoining or communicating with others; the vestibule of the ear.

- W -

WHITE NOISE: A composite of a wide range of frequencies, such as running water, which masks all speech sounds.

WITHDRAWAL: Termination of the administration of a habit-forming substance, and the physiological readjustment which takes place upon discontinuation.

RESOURCES

ALCOHOL

National Clearinghouse for Alcoholic Information
    PO Box 2345
    Rockville, MD 20852
    (301) 468-2600

Women for Sobriety
    PO Box 618
    Quakertown, PA 18951
    (215) 536-8026

ALLERGIES

Food Allergy Center
    53-31 Marathon Parkway
    Little Neck, NY 11362
    (800) YES-RELIEF

Society for Clinical Ecology
    PO Box 16106
    Denver, CO 80216
    (303) 622-9755

BOOKS

Cure for all Cancers, Hulda Regehr Clark, Ph.D., N.d.
Cure for all Diseases, Hulda Regehr Clark, Ph.D., N.d.
    Order books at (800) 231-1776

Natural Relief From Tinnitus, Paul Yanick, Jr., Ph.D.,
        Keats Publishing, Inc., New Canaan, Connecticut
        (Available in most health stores).

CANCER TREATMENT

American Biologics
    1180 Walnut Avenue
    Chula Vista, CA 92011

American Metabolic Institute
    416 W. San Ysidro Blvd.
    Suite L124
    San Ysidro, CA 92073

CHIROPRACTORS

Scott Calcaretta, DC
    862 Folsom St.
    San Francisco, CA 94107

Jacques J. Dezavelle, DC
    1118 Second St.
    Encinitas, CA 92024
    (619) 436-5151

Andrew W. Specht, DC
    230 Second Street, Suite 101
    Encinitas, CA 92024
    (619) 632-0098

William F. Wells, DC
    6565 Balboa Avenue, Suite A
    San Diego, CA 92111
    (619) 541-1440

172

DENTISTS

Before you have any dental work done, I strongly urge you to purchase the book Tooth Truth by Frank J. Jerome, D.D.S. We can no longer assume that dentists will do what is best for us.
Order from Promotion Publishers, (800) 231-1776.

Comprehensive Dental
     4403 Manchester Avenue, Suite 105
     Encinitas, CA 92024

Health Consciousness
     PO Box 550
     Oviedo, Florida 32765

Tijuana Dentistry
     Avenida Ocamp #1651
     Tijuana, B.C. Mexico
     011-526-685-4566
     (Board certified in California. Dental lab on site.)

The Toxic Element Research Foundation (TERF)
     PO Box 80
     Colorado Springs, CO 80901

Dr. Joaquin Zavala, DDS
     Edificio Constitucion
     Calle 3ra. No. 8116 Int. 201
     Tijuana, B.C. Mexico
     011-52-66-300011

The Mittelman Newsletter
     263 West End Ave. #2A
     New York, NY 10023

Bio-Probe Newsletter
 PO Box 580160
 Orlando, Florida 32858

DETOX CENTERS, CLINICS & FACILITIES

Check your local Yellow Pages for "Detoxification Centers"

DRUGS

National Clearinghouse for Drug Abuse Information
 5600 Fishers Lane
 Rockville, MD 20857
 (301) 443-6500
 (Offers list of 3000 treatment centers)

ENVIRONMENT

Citizens Against Toxic Sprays
 1385 Bailey Avenue
 Eugene, OR 97402

Friends of the Earth
 1045 Sansome Street
 San Francisco, CA 94111
 (415) 433-7373

Human Ecology Action League (HEAL)
 (also for allergies)
 PO Box 1369
 Evanston, IL 60204-1369
 (312) 864-0995

Nigra Enterprises
      5699 Kanan Road
      Agora, CA 91301-3358
      (818) 889-6877
      (Offers all types of environmental purification
      products)

HEARING AID PROBLEMS

(Agencies to contact)

Better Business Bureau (in your city)
      (Contact by phone or writing)

Bureau of Consumer Affairs (in your city)
      Department of Consumer Compliant and Protection
      re: Hearing Aid Dispensers (contact by phone)

State Board of Medical Examiners (in your state)
      Department for Complaints with Hearing Aids
      Contact by phone or write to the office in your state

National Hearing Aid Society
      Board of Certification
      20361 Middlebelt
      Livonia, Michigan 48152

Ombudsman
      Public Affairs Department
      Contact at any of your major radio or television
      broadcasting stations in your city.

HEARING PRODUCTS

Ambient Shapes, Inc.
>PO Box 5069
>Hickory, NC 28063
>
>Major credit cards 1-800-438-2244
>1997 price: $149.00; 30 day money back guarantee

Auditory Research
>PO Box 2828
>Los Angeles, CA 90078
>This company is no longer in business.

Bio Ear
>(Herbal ear drops)
>Alive & Alert
>31566 Railroad Canyon Road, Suite 2000
>Canyon Lake, CA 92587
>(909) 244-4888
>
>Signatures
>19465 Brennan Avenue
>Perris, CA 92599
>(800) 551-2846

BLF #20, EARS (Drops that stimulates blood supply to the nerves bringing relief)

X-WAX (drops for impacted earwax).

Both of the above available from:
Health Center for Better Living
>6189 Taylor Road
>Naples, FL 33942

Bobalee Originals Ear Candles (removes impacted earwax).
8577 Coachman Way
West Jordan, UT 84088-5509

Dr. John's Special Eardrops
Dr. John's Research
Department S-97
Box 637
Taylor, MI 48180

Ear-Planes (designed to minimize ear pain aloft)
House Ear Institute
2122 W. Third Street
Los Angeles, CA 90057

Also available from
Hammacher Schlemmer
(800) 543-3366

Ear Relaxer (Special pillow to relieve Tinnitus)
P.O. Box 90
Victor, WV 25938

Hal-Hen Co.
36-14 11th Street
Long Island, NY 11106
(718) 392-6020

Potentials Unlimited, Inc.
Department CA
P.O. Box 10058
Bradenton, FL 34282

Sleepwell Ear Stops
Sleep Shade Co.
PO Box 414
Richmond, CA 94807

SoundScreen® (A masker)
> Mature Wisdom
> P.O. Box 28
> Hanover, PA 17333-0028
> (800) 691-9222
>
> (TV & Telephone amplification: alarm clocks for the hard of hearing.)

Thunder 29 Ear Muff
> Safety & Supply Co.
> 595 North Columbia Blvd.
> Portland, OR 97217
> (503) 283-9500

Zee Medical Inc.
> P.O. Box 19527
> Irvine, CA 92713
> (714) 252-9500
> (800) 841-8417

HEARING INSTITUTIONS

Deafness Research Foundation
> 9 East 38th Street
> New York, NY 10016
> Voice/TDD: (212) 684-6556
> Voice/TDD: (800) 535-DEAF

Electromedical Research Institute
> 2301 North Collins, Suite 190
> Arlington, TX 76011
> (214) 354-6466

Meniere's Network
    2000 Church Street
    Box 111
    Nashville TN 37236
    (615) 329-7807

HEARING AND TINNITUS
ASSOCIATIONS

American Tinnitus Association (ATA)
    PO Box 5
    Portland, OR 97207
    (502) 248-9985

Association of Holistic Healing Centers
    2100 Mediterranean Avenue #40
    Virginia Beach, VA 23451
    (804) 498-2598

Ear Research Foundation
    1921 Floyd Street
    Sarasota, FL 34239

Hearing Education and Awareness for Rockers
    H.E.A.R.
    (415) 773-9590

Self-Help for Hard of Hearing People, Inc.
    7800 Wisconsin Avenue
    Bethesda, MD 20814
    (301) 657-2248

The Hyperacusis Network
>Dan Malcone, Editor
>120 Traders Point Lane
>Green Bay, WI 54302
>HOME: (414) 468-4663
>FAX: (414) 432-3321
>(Free quarterly publication. Donations   accepted.)

Occupational Hearing Services
>PO Box 1880
>Media, PA 19063

HERBS AND HERB TEAS

Arizona Natural Products
>8281 East Evans Road #105
>Scottsdale, AZ 85260
>(602) 991-4414

Health Fest
>74 20th Street
>Brooklyn, NY 11232

Nature's Sunshine Products
>PO Box 1000
>Spanish Fork, UT 84660

Nighty Night
>Traditional Medicinals
>4515 Ross Road
>Sebastopol, CA 95472

Swiss Labs, Inc.
>405 N. Palm Canyon Drive
>Palm Springs, CA 92262

HOLISTIC HEALTH

Association for Holistic Health
PO Box 9532
San Diego, CA 92109
(619) 275-2694

American Holistic Medical Association
6932 Little River Turnpike
Annandale, VA 22003
(703) 642-5880

Holisatic Horizons
PO Box 2868
Oakland, CA 94618

Ronald Jahner, N.D., C.A. (Montana)
13983 Mango Dr., Suite 206
Del Mar, CA 92014

HYPERACTIVITY

Feingold Association of the United States
PO Box 6550
Alexandria, VA 22306

MASSAGE

American Massage & Therapy Association
PO Box 1270
Kingsport, TN 37662
(615) 245-8071

MEDICAL DOCTORS

Soraya Hoover, MD
150 W. Parker #705
Houston, TX 77076

John W. House
Otologic Medical Group, Inc.
2122 W. Third Street
Los Angeles, CA 90057

Michael Klaper, M.D.
2611 Vanderbilt, Suite 2
Redondo Beach, CA 90278

John J. Shea, MD
Shea Clinic
1060 Madison Avenue
Memphis, TN 38104

NATURAL HYGIENE BOOKS

Dick Gregory's Natural Diet for Folks Who Eat:
Cookin' with Mother Nature
Harper & Row, Publishers
New York, Hagerstown, San Francisco

Karen Cross Whyte: ORIGINAL DIET
Troubador Press San Francisco

Raw Energy
Leslie and Susannah Kenton
Warner Books, Inc.
666 Fifth Avenue
New York, NY 10103

182

The Uncook Book
        Elizabeth & Dr. Elton Baker
        Communication Creativity
        PO Box 213
        Saguache, CO 81149

NOTE: All of the above books are out of print. They can be found in used book stores.

NATURAL HYGIENE
ORGANIZATIONS

The American Natural Hygiene Society, Inc.
        PO Box 30630
        Tampa, FL 33630

Get Well * Stay Well, America!
        Attn: Victoria Bidwell
        1776 Hygiene Joy Way
        Mt. Vernon, WA 98273
        (206) 428-3687
        (Provides a catalog of natural hygien books)

Health Excellence Systems
        See Life Science Institute

Hygienic Community Network
        2732 W. College Street
        Springfield, MO 65802
        (417) 831-3188

Life Science
        1108 Regal Row
        Manchaca, TX 78162

Life Science Institute
    2929 W. Anderson Lane
    Austin, TX 78757
    (800) 889-9989

Natural Hygience, Inc.
    Attn: Jo Willard
    PO Box 2123
    Huntington, CT 06484
    (203) 929-1557

Orkos Institute
    584 Castro Street
    San Francisco, CA 94114

NATURAL HYGIENE
RETREATS

Abunda Life Health Hotel & Clinic
    208 Third Avenue
    Asbury Park, NY 07712

Alternative Therapy Center
    Dr. Bernarr Zovluck
    683 S. McCadden Place
    Los Angeles, CA 90005
    (213) 931-7201
    (Offers health consultations, healing, nutritional
    guidance, fitness training, body work, lectures,
    publications)

American Living Fopod Health Recovery Center
    1147 E. Broadway #118
    Glendale, CA 91205
    (818) 952-4940

Ann Wigmore Foundation
196 Commonwealth Avenue
Boston, MA 02116
(617) 266-6955

Ann Wigmore Foundation
2417 W. Lincoln Avenue
Montebello, CA 90640
(213) 723-1994

Club Hygiene
105 Bruce Court
Marathon, FL 33050
(305) 743-3168

Creative Health Institute
918 Union City Road
Union City, MI 49094
(517) 278-6260

Ricki D. Grunberg, MA, MsT
(offers private counseling)
P.O. Box 3473
Madison, WI 53704
(608) 257-2144

Health Oasis
Route 2, PO Box 10
Tilly, AR 72679
(501) 496-2364

Helena Henn
3990 Hillview Road
Santa Maria, CA 93455
(805) 934-3614

Hippocrates Health Institute
　　　1443 Palmdale Court
　　　West Palmdale, FL 33441
　　　(407) 471-8876

Hygeia Health Retreat
　　　439 East Main Street
　　　Yorktown, TX 78164
　　　(512) 564-3670

Nature's First Law
　　　P.O. Box 900202
　　　San Diego, CA 92190
　　　(800) 205-2350

Optimum Health Institute of San Diego
　　　(formerly Hippocrates West)
　　　6970 Central Avenue
　　　Lemon Grove, CA 92045
　　　(619) 464-3346

Pawling Health Manor
　　　PO Box 401
　　　Hyde Park, NY 12538
　　　(914) 889-4141

Scott's Natural Health Institute
　　　PO Box 361095
　　　Strongsville, Ohio 44136
　　　(216) 238-6930

NOISE

Acoustical Society of America
335 East 45th Street
New York, NY 10017

Citizens Against Noise
2729 West Lunt Avenue
Chicago, IL 60645

OSTEOPATHIC COLLEGES

I no longer list most osteopath colleges because their curriculums have been changed to conform to the requirements of allopathic medicne.

American Academy of Osteopathy
(Contact for an osteopath in your area)
3500 De Pauw Blvd., Suite 1080
Indianapolis, IN 45268-1136
(317) 879-1881

REFLEXOLOGY

Better Health With Foot Reflexology:
The Original Ingham Method
by Dwight C. Byers
Ingham Publishing, Inc.
Saint Petersburg, FL

Hand Reflexology: Key to Perfect Health
by Mildred Carter
Parker Publishing Company, Inc.
West Nyack, NY
(Can be found in libraries, Reference No. 615.822)

International Institute of Reflexology
Ingham Publishing, Inc.
5650 1st Avenue North
St. Petersburg, FL 33733
(813) 343-4811

F.R.A.A.
    A Non Profit Corp.
    P.O. Box 7622
    Mission Hills, CA 91346-7622

SMOKING

Five-Day Plan to Stop Smoking*
    Seventh-Day Adventist Church
    Narcotics Education Division
    6840 Eastern Ave. NW
    Washington, DC 20012
    (202) 723-0800

*I recommend this nonsectarian program.

Also check your local phone book for:

American Heart Association
American Lung Association
Schick Laboratories
SmokeEnders

VEGETARIAN

Club Veg (A newsletter that tells of vegetarian activities)
    5663 Balboa Avenue #334
    San Diego, CA 92111
    (619) 282-3900
    (send S.A.S.E. for a sample newsletter.)

Club Veg of San Diego
    3716 35th St.
    San Diego, CA 92104

Jewish Vegetarian Society
    PO Box 5722
    Baltimore, MD 21208
    (301) 486-4948

Live Food Singles Club - World Wide
    11015 Cumpston Street
    North Hollywood, CA 91601
    (818) 763-1000

North American Vegetarianism Society
    PO Box 72
    Dolgeville, NY 13329

The Rawsome News
    Raw Food Support Group of San Diego County
    Box 4766
    San Diego, CA 92164-4766
    (Send S.A.S.E. for a sample newsletter).

San Francisco Vegetarian Society, Inc.
    1450 Broadway, No. 4
    San Francisco, CA 94109
    (415) 775-6874

Vegetarian Information Service, Inc.
    PO Box 5888
    Bethesda, MD 20814
    (301) 530-1737

Vegetarian Society, Inc.
    PO Box 34427
    Los Angeles, CA 90034
    (213) 281-1907

SPECIAL MENTION

The Essene Gospel of Peace
  (about Jesus and fasting)
  IBS International
  PO Box 205
  Matsqui, British Columbia
  Canada VOX 1SO

or from

The Gerston Institute
  PO Box 430
  Bonita, CA 91908

Why Christians Get Sick
  Rev. George H. Malkmus
  Hallelujah Acres Publishing
  122 E. Main Street
  Rogersville, TN 37857
  (615)-272-7800

REFERENCES

1. Marshall Cavendish, Illustrated Encyclopedia of Family Health, London and New York, 1983, 6:665.
2. The People's Medical Manual, Doubleday and Co. Inc. Garden City, New York, 1986, p535.
3. Lawrence Lamb, MD The Health Letter, Report 51, PO Box 787, Gibbstown, New Jersey, P2.
4. Arthur S. Freese, MD, You and Your Hearing, Charles Scribner's Sons, New York, 1979, p119.
5. Wyngaarden and Smith, Cecil Textbook of Medicine, W. B. Saunders Co., Philadelphia, 1985, 23:2040.
6. J. I. Rodale, The Encyclopedia of Common Diseases, Rodale Books, Inc., Emmaus, Pennsylvania, 1973, p32.
7. American Tinnitus Association, PO Box 5, Portland, OR 97207, 11:3, Sept. 1986, p7.
   a. 12:4, 1987, p1.
   b. 12:4, 1987, pp 1 & 5.
   c. 12:1, March 1987, p4.
   d. 12:3, September 1987, p4.
   e. 11:2, June 1986, p2.
   f. 11:3, September 1986, p3.
   g. Information About Tinnitus (Head Noises), Pamphlet.
   h. 11:4, December 1986, p2.
   i. 13:1, March 1988, p7.
   j. 11:4, December 1986, p1.
   k. 11:4, December 1986, p3.
8. The Book of Health, Franklin Watts, New York, London, Toronto, 1981, pp550-551.

9.   Fishbein's Illustrated Medical and Health
     Encyclopedia, H. S. Stuttman, Inc., Westport,
     Connecticut, 1981, 16:2131-2132.
10. R. D. Berendt and E. L. Charles, Quieting: A
     Practical Guide to Noise Control, US Dept. of
     Commerce, July 1976, p8.
11. G. Dekle Taylor, MD, "Acoustic Trauma in the
     Sports Hunter," Laryngoscope, Feb. 1966,
     76:863-879.
12. Richard Carmen, MD, Our Endangered
     Hearing, Understanding & Coping with
     Hearing Loss, Rodale Press, Emmaus, PA, 1977,
     p36.
13. Jack Vernon, MD, "Tinnitus: a legal problem
     with a familiar ring, "Oregon State Bar Bulletin,
     Oct. 1983, p.
14. Leigh Silverman, "Loud Music & Hearing Loss,"
     Audio, 73:1, DOI Haghette Publishers, Inc.,
     New York, Jan. 1989, p76.
15. Haraldsson, PO and Bergstedt, M.,
     "Unconsciousness and Persistent Tinnitus
     Caused by Lighting Injury to the Ear During
     Telephoning," Lakartidningen, 80:2024, 1983.
16. Debra Lynn Dadd, Nontoxic & Natural,
     Jeremy P. Tarcher, Inc., Los Angeles, 1984.
17. Walter E. Rahm, Jr., et al, "The Effects of
     Anesthetics Upon the Ear," Annals Otol Rhinol
     Laryngol, 1962, pp16-123.
18. E. Mindell, MD, Earl Mindell's Vitamin Bible,
     Rawson Wade Pub., New York, 1979, p213.
19. Paavo Airola, PhD, ND, How To Get Well
     Health Plus Publishers, PO Box 22001, Phoenix,
     AZ 85028, 1974, pp31-32.
     a.   Are You Confused?, pp93-103.

20. Roger J. Williams, <u>Nutrition Against Disease</u>, Pitman Publishing Corp., New York, Toronto, 1971, p168.
21. J. T. Cooper, MD, with Paul Hagan, <u>Dr. Cooper's Fabulous Fructose Diet</u>, M. Evans and Co., Inc., New York, p124.
22. Ross Fishman, PhD, <u>The Encyclopedia of Psychoactive Drugs, Alcohol: and Alcoholism</u>, Solomon H. Snyder, MD, Editor, Chelsa House Pub., New York, New Haven, Philadelphia, 1986, p42.
    a. <u>Marijuana: Its Effects on Mind & Body</u>, Mariam Cohen, PhD, pp59-67.
    b. <u>Cocaine: A New Epidemic</u>, Chris-Ellyn Johnson, PhD, pp32-37.
    c. <u>Prescription Narcotics: The Addictive Painkillers</u>, Paul R. Sanberg, PhD, and Michael D. Bunsey, pp39-47 and pp66-77.
23. Phyllis Saifer, MD, and Merla Zellerbach, <u>Detox</u>, Jeremy P. Tarcher, Inc., Los Angeles, 1984, pp118-119.
24. <u>Better Homes and Gardens New Family Medical Guide</u>, Meredith Corp., Des Moines, Iowa, 1982, p288.
25. C. Fry, "Why Do Antibiotics Prevent Infection?" <u>Health Scene Newsletter</u>, 1:6, pp3-4 (undated). Health Excellence Systems, 1108 Regal Row, PO Box 609, Manchaca, TX 78652.
    a. <u>Are You A Candidate for Cancer?</u>, Herbert Shelton, MD.
    b. <u>Medical Drugs on Trial--Verdict Guilty</u>, Sidhwa.
    c. T. C. Fry, <u>Health Reporter</u>, 1:8, p27.
    d. T. C. Fry, "The Myth of Health in American," pamphlet #C-811-M.

e. John Oliver, <u>Health Reporter</u>, 1:1, pp22 & 27.

f. Herbert M. Shelton, MD & William L. Esser, MD, "Migraine Headache," pamphlet (no number).

g. Vicky Bidwell, "Objections to the StandardAmerican Diet," <u>Healthful Living</u>, 4:3, 1985 p23.

h. Herbert M. Shelton, MD "Fasting as the Quickest Way to Overcome Disease," <u>Health Reporter</u>, 1:2, (not dated) p7.

i. Marti Wheeler, <u>Health Reporter</u>, 1:19, p4.

j. Chester P. Yozwick, NA, "Allergies,' A World Without Love," <u>Health Reporter</u>, 1:18, pp20-21.

k. T. C. Fry, <u>Health Reporter</u>, 1:18, p15.

l. T. C. Fry, <u>Health Reporter</u>, 1:18, p1.

m. Herbert M. Shelton, MD, <u>Health Reporter</u>, 1:18 p2.

n. T. C. Fry, <u>Health Reporter</u>, 1:18, p15.

o. Herbert M. Shelton, MD, "Overcoming Diabetes," pamphlet (no number).

p. T. C. Fry, "How Do You Deal With Mèniére's Disease?, '<u>The Healthway Advisor</u>, (not dated), 1:6, p8.

q. E. McBean, PhD, ND, <u>Vaccinations Do Not Protect and Court Violates Federal Law In Vaccination Case</u>.

r. T. C. Fry, <u>Health Reporter</u>, 1:7, p17.

s. Marti Fry, <u>Health Reporter</u>, 1:12, p24.

t. T. C. Fry, <u>Health Reporter</u>, 1:8, pp26-27.

u. Herbert M. Shelton, MD, <u>Health Reporter</u>, 1:8, p2.

    v.   Susan Hazard, PhD, <u>Health Reporter</u>,
           1:16, pp26-27.
    w. T. C. Fry, <u>Health Reporter</u>, 1:1, p28.
    x.   Marti Fry, <u>Health Reporter</u>, 1:2, p6.
    y.   <u>T. C. Fry, Health Reporter</u>, 1:7, p16.
    z.   <u>T. C. Fry, Health Reporter</u>, 1:4, p16.

26. Roger R. Reddel, et al, "Ototoxicity In Patients Receiving Cisplatin: Importance of Dose and Method of Drug Administration," <u>Cancer Treatment Reports</u>, 66:1, Jan 1982, pp19-23.

27. Virginia Livingston-Wheeler, MD, Edmond G. Addeo, <u>The Conquest of Cancer</u>, Franklin Watts, New York, London, 1984, pp40, 40-46.

28. Edith Efron, <u>The Apocalyptics: Cancer and the Big Lie: How Environmental Politics Controls What We Know About Cancer</u>, Simon and Schuster, New York, 1984.

29. Ruth Winter, <u>A Consumer's Dictionary of Cosmetic Ingredients</u>, Crown Pub., Inc., New York, 1974.

30. Michele McCormick, <u>Designer-Drug Abuse</u>, An Impact Book, New York, London, 1989, pp12-60.

31. <u>Understanding Human Behavior</u>, Columbia House, New York 1974, 5:531.

32. Vern Modeland, "When Bells Are Ringing (But There Aren't Any Bells)," <u>FDA Consumer</u>, Dept. of Health and Human Services, 5600 Fischers Lane, Rockville, MD 20857, (April 1989), pp9-12.

33. M. S. Pathy, "The Use, Action and Side Effects of Diuretics," <u>Gerontal. Clin.</u>, 1971, 13:261-268.

34. Paul Yanick, Jr., PhD, "Nutrition Can Help Your Hearing," <u>Let's Live</u>, 444 Larchmont Boulevard, Los Angeles, CA 90004, May 1981, pp42-45.

35. N. Pritikin, <u>The Pritikin Permanent Weight-Loss Manual</u>, Grosset & Dunlap, New York, 1981, p16.

36. Dennis McFadden, <u>Tinnitus: Facts, Theories, and Treatments</u>, National Academy Press, Washington, DC, 1982, p62.

37. Michael J. Kraemer, MD, et al, "Risk Factors for Persistent Middle-Ear Effusions," <u>Journal of American Medical Association</u>, Feb. 25, 1983, 249:8, pp1022-1025.

38. John Waldrop and Janice McCall Failes, <u>Natural Health and Wellness Encyclopedia</u>, FC&A Publishing, 103 Clover Green, Peachtree City, Georgia, 30269, p257.

39. S. S. Field, "Nicotine: Profile of Peril," <u>Reader's Digest</u>, Pleasantville, New York, 10570, Sept. 1973, pp77-80.

40. <u>Earl Mindell's Pill Bible</u>, Bantam Books, Toronto, New York, 1984, pp306-307.

41. American Lung Association of San Diego and Imperial Counties, 2750 Fourth Ave., San Diego, CA 92103, (619) 297-3901.

42. Water Test Corp., Scytheville Row, PO Box 186, New London, NH 03257, Jan. 1985, pamphlet.

43. M. Cline, <u>The Junk Food Withdrawal Manual</u>, The Nutri-Books Corp., Box 5793, Denver, CO 80217.

44. Robert S. Mendelsohn, <u>Confessions of a Medical Heretic</u>, Contemporary Books, Inc., Chicago, 1979, p39.

45. <u>Black's Medical Dictionary</u>, Wm A. R. Thomson, MD (ed), 33rd Edition, Butler and Tanner Ltd., Frome and London, 1981, p743.

46. Isadore Rosenfeld, MD, <u>Modern Prevention: The New Medicine</u>, THE LINDEN PRESS/Simon and Schuster, New York, 1986, p260.
47. W. E. Rahm, "The Effects of Anesthesia on the Ear," <u>Annals Oto Rhinol Laryngol</u>, 1962, pp16-23.
48. Jane E. Brody, "Letting Fever Run Its Course," <u>New York Times</u>, December 28, 1982, Section III, 1:1.
49. Margie Garrison, <u>I Cured My Arthritis: You Can Too</u>, 10 Witherel, Suite 32, Detroit, MI 48226, (313) 963-2728. (self-published).
50. John Yudkin, MD, <u>Sweet and Dangerous</u>, Peter H. Wyden, Inc., New York,   1 9 7 2 , pp110-121.
51. E. M. Abrahamson, MD & A. W. Pezet, <u>Body, Mind & Sugar</u>, Avon Books, New York, 1977, pp176-195.
52. William Dufty, <u>Sugar Blues</u>, Warner Books, Co., New York, 1975.
53. J. I. Rodale, <u>Natural Health, Sugar and the Criminal Mind</u>, Pyramid Books, 919 Third Ave., New York, 10022, 1968.
54. Usoa Busto, MD, <u>New England Journal of Medicine</u>, 315:14, Oct. 2, 1986, pp854-859.
55. J. Russell Sneddon, M.D., M.B.N.O.A., <u>How to Cure Catarrhal Deafness and Head Noises</u>, Health for All Publishing Company, Gateway House, Bedford Park, Croydon CR92AT, Surrey, England.
56. <u>Van Nostrand Reinhold Encyclopedia of Chemistry</u>, Fourth Edition, Douglass M. Considine, PE, Editor-in-Chief, Van Nostrand Reinhold Co., New York, Cincinnati, 1984, pp115-116.

57. Arnold R. Saslow, Dr. Ph., Mph, and Paul S. Clark, "Carbon Monoxide Poisoning," Journal of Occupational Medicine, 15:490-493, 1983.
58. Insight, Washington, DC, Oct 1, 1990, pp48-49.
59. Hal A. Huggins, DDS, It's All In Your Head, PO Box 2589, Colorado Springs, CO, 80901.
60. Joyal Taylor, DDS, The Complete Guide to Mercury Toxicity From Dental Fillings, Scripps Publishing, San Diego, CA, 1988, pp76-77.
61. C. Edmonds, "Hearing Loss with Frequent Diving (deaf divers)," Undersea Biomedical Research, 12:3, Sept. 1985, pp315-318.
62. Michael I. Weintraub, MD, "High-Impact Aerobic Exercises and Vertigo--A Possible Cause of Bilateral Vestibulopathy," New England Journal of Medicine, 323:23, Dec. 6, 1990, p1633.
63. Janice McCall Failes and Frank W. Cawood, Natural Healing Encyclopedia, FC&A Publishing, Peachtree City, GA 30296, pp74-75.
64. J. U. Toglia, MD, et al, "Vestibular and Audiological Aspects of Whiplash Injury and Head Trauma," Journal of Forensic Sciences, 14:219-226, 1969.
65. Charles B. Clayman, MD, (Ed), The American Medical Association Encyclopedia of Medicine, Random House, New York, 1989, p113.
66. Marshall Mandell, MD, and Theron G. Randolph, Dr. Mandell's 5-Day Allergy Relief System, Harper & Row Publishing Inc., New York, 1978.
67. K. Thomsen, et al, "Glomus jugulare tumors," J. Laryngol Otol., 1975, 89:113-1121.

68. John Poppy, "What's the Buzz?" Esquire, 1790 Broadway, New York, 10019, April 1989, pp77-79.
69. James Kawchak, MD, Journal of Occupational Medicine, 3:1, 1963.
70. B. H. Senturia, MD, Laryngoscope 57:633-656.
71. Abraham Schulman et al., Tinnitus: Diagnosis/Treatment, Lea & Febeger, Philadelphia, 1991.
72. Dan Malcore, The Hyperacusis Network, 120 Traders Point Lane, Green Bay, WI 54302. Sep. 1992, Dec. 1992, and Supplement issues.
73. Helping Your Health With Pointed Pressure Therapy, Parker Publishing Company, Inc., West Nyack, NY, p. 187.
74. Andrew P. Freeland, MD, Deafness: The Facts, Oxford University Press, 1989, pp66-67.
75. Otolaryngology, 70; 79:992.
76. Ann. Otol. Rhino. Laryngo., 58; 67: 185 L.C.
77. Athero., 85; 55 (3); 267-81.
78. Family Medical Guide, William Marrow and Company, Inc., New York, 1983, p339.
79. The Encyclopedia Britannica, The Encyclopedia Britannica Co., Publishers, New York, 1911, 23:129.
80. Carty Stern, "Do You Lose Your Balance?", Parade Magazine, Parade Publications, Inc., 750 Third Avenue, New York, 10017, Aug. 2, 1987, p16.
81. James T. Spencer, MD, "Hyperlipoproteinemias In The Etiology of Inner Ear Disease," Laryngoscope, 5:639-678, May, 1973.
82. M. Coleman Harris, MD, F.A.C.P., et al., Practical Allergy, F.A. Davis Company, Philadelphia, p279.

83. Patricia R. House, et al, <u>CIBA Foundation Symposium 85</u>, Pitman Books Ltd., London, 1981, pp193-198.

84. John J. Shea, MD, et al, "Medical Treatment of Tinnitus," Presented at the meeting of the American Otological Society, Inc., Vancouver, British Columbia, May 9-10, 1981. Reprints--John J. Shea, Shea Clinic, 1060 Madison Ave., Memphis TN 38104.

85. Louise L. Hay, <u>You Can Heal Your Life</u>, Hay House, Santa Monica, CA 1987.

86. Herbert Benson, <u>The Relaxation Response</u>, Morrow, New York, 1975.

87. M. B. Lubin, MD, "TMJ Syndrome," <u>Carlsbad Magazine</u>, 2945 Harding Street, Suite 211, Carlsbad, CA pp32-33.

88. Dixie Farley, TM Disorders: "Aches and Pains from Flaws in the Jaws," <u>FDA Consumer</u>, Office of Public Affairs 5600 Fisher's Lane, Rockville, MD 20857, (301) 443-3220, June 1988, pp7-9.

89. Jack Alpan, DDS, Dental Health Center Newsletter, 2440 W. 3rd Street, Los Angeles, CA (213) 383-3833, Dec. 1979.

90. Andrew Kaplan, DMD, "Self-Help for TMJ," <u>Prevention</u>, Emmaus PA, Nov. 1988, pp46-54. Reprinted with permission from <u>The TMJ Book</u>, by Kaplan and Gray Williams, Jr., Pharos Books, New York, 1988.

91. James Dillon, <u>TMJ, The Self Help Program</u>, Surrey Park Press, 1990.

92. Hallowell, David, MD, and S. RichardSilverman, PhD, <u>Hearing and Deafness</u>, 3rd Edition, Holt, Renehart and Winston, New York, Chicago, 1970, pp120-

122.93.
93. George E. Urban, Jr., MD, "Severe Sensorineural Hearing Loss Associated with Viral Hepatitis, "Southern Medical Journal, June 1978, 71:6, pp724-725.
94. Harris L. Coulter, PhD, Vaccination, Social Violence and Criminology: The Medical Assault on the American Brain, Str Emp Med, 1990.
95. Brian Inglis & Ruth West, The Alternative Health Guide, Alfred A. Knopf, New York, 1983, p133.
96. N. J. Marks, MD, et al, "A controlled trial of acupuncture in tinnitus," The Journal of Laryngology and Otology, Nov. 1984, 98:1103-1109.
97. Nathaniel Altman, The Chiropractic Alternative, J. P. Tarcher, Inc., Los Angeles, CA 1981, pp21-22.
98. The Alternative Newsletter, Mountain Home Publishers, July 1991, 4:1, p8.
99. Victoria Bidwell, 1776 The Hygiene Joy Way, Mount Vernon, WA 98273, (206) 428-3687.
100. Ito J. Sakakihara, "Suppression of Tinnitus by Coclear Implantation," Am J Otolaryngol, 1994 Mar-Apr; 15(2):145-8
101. Robert W. Baloh, Dizziness, Hearing Loss and Tinnitus, F. A. Davis Co., Philadelphia, 1984, pp172-174.
102. Inge Dougans with Suzanne Ellis, REFLEXOLOGY foot massage for total health, Element Inc., publishers, Rockport, MA, 1991, p17.
103. Leon Chaitow, ND, DO, Alternative Therapies: A Complete Health-Care System, Thorsons Publishers Limited, Wellingborough,

Northamptonshire, 1985, p17.
104. W. I. Acton, "The Effects of Industrial Airborne Ultrasound on Humans," Ultrasonics, 12:124-128, 1974. (The author is at the University of Southampton, UK)
105. W. I. Acton, "Exposure to Industrial Ultrasound: Hazards Appraisal and Control," J. Soc. Occup.Med., 33:107-113, 1983.
106. Richard Carmen and Dion Svihovec, "Tinnitus Treatment by Relaxation and/or Biofeedback," AUDIOLOGY in Practice, 111(2):6-7, 1986.
107. Paul Yanick, Jr., PhD, "Tinnitus--a Holistic Approach," Hearing Instruments, 1981, 32:7, p13.
108. Deepak Chopra, MD, "Magical Mind, Magical Body," (six audio cassettes), Nightingale-Conant Corporation, 7300 North Lehigh Avenue, Chicago Ill 60648, (1991 price $59.95 plus shipping and tax).
109. Alan H. Nittler, MD, A New Breed of Doctor, Pyramid House, New York, 1972, p95.
110. Arnold Ehret, Arnold Ehret's Mucusless-Diet Healing System, Ehret Literature Publishing Co., Inc., Dobbs Ferry, NY 10522, pp15-24.
111. Sheila Shea, "Colon Irrigation," flyer, Basic Health Institute, 330 Fourth Avenue, San Diego, CA 92103.
112. Gary N. Lewkovich, DC, Colonic Therapy, Self published San Marcos, CA 92069, pp1-4.
113. Rob*ert Grey, The Colon Health Handbook, Emerald Publishers, PO Box 11830, Reno, NV 89510.
114. Jason Winter, In Search of the Perfect Cleanse, Vinton Publishing, 4055 S.

Spencer, Suite 245, Las Vegas, NV 89109.
115. Abraham Shulman, "Vasodilator-antihistamine Therapy and Tinnitus Control," Journal of Laryngol. Oto. (Suppl): 102-106, 1981.
116. Durk Pearson and Sandy Shaw, Life Extension: A Practical Scientific Approach, Warner Books, New York, 1982, pp126-131.
117. Prevention Magazine, April 1992, p54.
118. Hyperacusis Network, December 1992, p7.
119. George E. Shambaugh, Jr., MD, "Zinc for Tinnitus, Imbalance, and Hearing Loss in the Elderly", The American Journal of Otology, 7:6, Nov. 1986.
120. Cherie Calbom and Maureen Keane, Juicing for Life, Avery Publishing Group Inc., Garden City Park, New York, 1992, p264.
121. Severn L. Schaeffer, "An Introduction to Anopsology," 25 Rue Des Longs-Pres, 92100 Boulonge, France, 1985.
122. Jonathan Palmer, "The Health Breakthrough of the Century Part I," CTC Health Letter #1, PO Box 2853, Scottsdale, AZ 85252, p6.

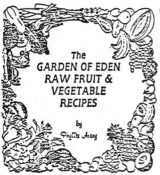

THE GARDEN OF EDEN RAW FRUIT & VEGETABLE RECIPES
by Phyllis Avery

(all vegan—no milk products)

FRUIT RECIPES:

HORS D'OEUVRES, FRUIT DISHES, FRUIT SYRUPS, FRUIT SHAKES (includes banana "ice cream") and FRUIT DRINKS!

VEGETABLE RECIPES:

HORS D'OEUVRES, SOUPS, DIPS, DRESSINGS (made without vinegar, mayonnaise, or oil), and 50 MAIN DISHES.

The 126-page book also offers an introduction to natural hygiene (the eating of raw food), a two-page food combining chart and basic food-combining principles, a chapter on selecting and storing fruits and vegetables, and a list of natural hygiene organizations.

The recipes conform to the principles of natural hygiene.

Retail price — $10.95.

Shipping -- $1.75. California add 7.75% sales tax.

GetWell ★ StayWell, America! ... joyfully presents ...
The Health Seekers' YearBook

A Revolutionist's HandBook for Getting Well & Staying Well without The Medicine Men
...With A Whole-Hearted and Enthusiastic, Full Endorsement and Foreword
From Dr. V.V. Vetrano - One of the World's Foremost Authorities on Natural Hygiene!

PARTIAL LIST OF SUBJECTS

CHAPTER ONE

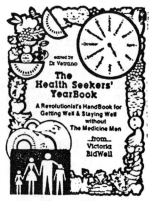

*The 4 Best Reasons Not to
  Take Drugs
*The 3 Lifestyle Causes of
  Disease
*The One Cause of All Disease
*The Seven Stages of Disease
*Enhance Your Immune System

CHAPTER TWO

*How to Detoxify The Body
*Fasting Is NOT Starvation
*Fasting in Chronic Disease
*Who Should Fast
*Who Should Not Fast

CHAPTER THREE

*Exercise and The Ideal Diet Build Health
*Stretching: Unique Features and Benefits
*Aerobics
*Weight Training
*Exercise Log

CHAPTER FOUR

*Physical, Physiolocical, Emotional,
  Mental, and Spiritual Health
*The Tell-Tale Signs of Depression
*Taming the Compulsive Personality
*The Addiction Syndrome
*The Life-Events Stress Test
*The 5 Stages of Burnout
*The Psychology of Low Self Esteem
*Exercise As a Positive Addiction
*Alcohol Withdrawal and Detoxification
*Nicotine Withdrawal
*The 7 Stages of Denial

CHAPTER 9

*Menus for the Entire Year

CHAPTER 10

*Special Recipes
  Dressing Recipes
*Morning Meals for Kids
*Brown-Bag Recipes

CHAPTER 11

*Seven Main Holiday Menus

CHAPTER 12

*An Expose on the Exorbitant Cost of Eating
  the Standard American Diet
*Health Costs and Diet
*Four Arguments for the Elimination of
  Television

CHAPTER 13

*365 Thought Provoking Quotes about Food

CHAPTER 14

*Sources
  Dehydrated Vegetable Seasoning
  The Body Slant
  Hygienic Retreats
  Hygenic Doctors
  Organic Food Outlets

460 PAGES!
Only $25 + shipping

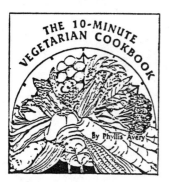

THE 10-MINUTE VEGETARIAN COOKBOOK

By Phyllis Avery

Phyllis offers the harried meal preparer quick, nutritious dishes that are steamed from 4 to 10 minutes. The main ingredient in all of the recipes are fresh vegetables. All recipes are entrees. The soups and salads are hearty enough for a complete meal. No-nonsense recipes -- all ingredients are common items, with minimal use of processed foods.

The peeling and chopping of vegetables can be shared by the whole family, making preparation time even shorter.

The 143-page book offers 192 recipes.

Retail price -- $11.95

Shipping -- $1.75. California add 7.75% sales tax.

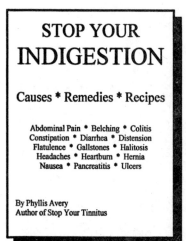

STOP YOUR
INDIGESTION

Causes * Remedies * Recipes

Abdominal Pain * Belching * Colitis
Constipation * Diarrhea * Distension
Flatulence * Gallstones * Halitosis
Headaches * Heartburn * Hernia
Nausea * Pancreatitis * Ulcers

By Phyllis Avery
Author of Stop Your Tinnitus

STOP YOUR INDIGESTION

Causes, Remedies, Recipes

By Phyllis Avery

You can be over your indigestion within 24 hours and never suffer from it again!

The second section offers easy, natural ways to overcome such problems as abdominal pain, belching, colitis, constipation, diarrhea, distention, flatulence, gallstones, halitosis, headaches, heartburn, hernia, nausea, pancreatitis, ulcers and many other problems that arise from failure to digest food.

The third section deals with selecting foods that are compatible in digestive chemistry with some typical recipes. The book also includes a resource list and a glossary.

Retail price -- $14.95

Shipping -- $1.75. California add 7.75% sales tax.

HELP FOR TINNITUS

I sent you a letter telling you of my problem, ear soreness and tinnitus, and I asked if you could help me, because the famous eye-ear-throat specialists I'd been to couldn't. However, they charged me $75, and told me to "live with it."

I heard from you very quickly. That alone meant a great deal to me (just someone giving a darn).

You sent me "Tinnitus and Other Hearing Problems" by Howard C. Long.

I have been doing as he suggested: niacin, then _lying on a slant board_, plus other vitamins. _In two days there is an improvement_ and I can't begin to tell you how grateful I am.

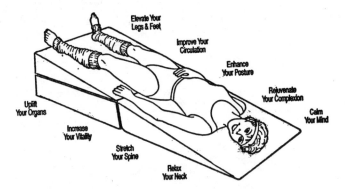

Elevate Your Legs & Feet
Improve Your Circulation
Enhance Your Posture
Rejuvenate Your Complexion
Calm Your Mind
Uplift Your Organs
Increase Your Vitality
Stretch Your Spine
Relax Your Neck

QUANTITY	PRODUCT	COST	SHIPPING	*CALIF TAX	TOTAL
	NEWTON BODYSLANT	165 EA.	**15.00 EA	*12.79 EA	$
	NAVY BEIGE GRAY BROWN GREEN FUCHSIA MAUVE BLACK			CHOOSE COLOR:	

*7.75% Sales Tax Applicable on CA orders only. Please allow 8-12 days delivery.
**Orders shipped by UPS. Please use street address only; NO P.O. BOX numbers.
Shipping to HI-AK-CAN-PR: $18.00

CHECK	
M/C	
VISA	NO._____ EXP. DATE_____

NAME_____ PHONE (___)_____

ADDRESS_____APT_____

CITY_____STATE____ ZIP_____